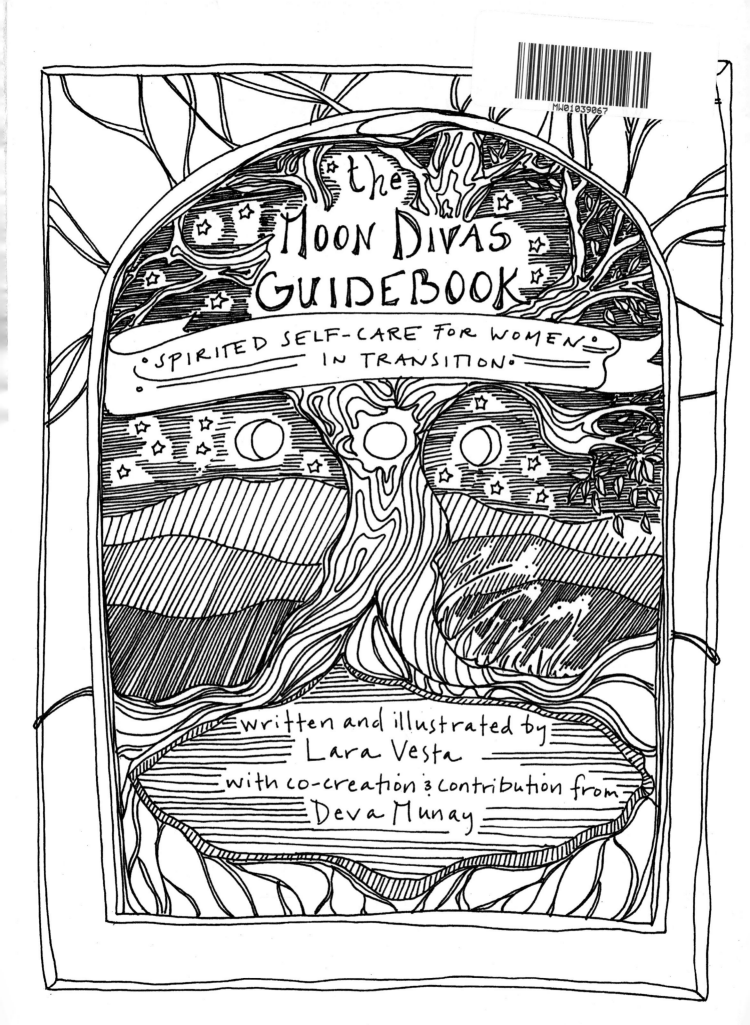

the
MOON DIVAS
GUIDEBOOK
· SPIRITED SELF-CARE FOR WOMEN ·
· IN TRANSITION ·

written and illustrated by
Lara Vesta
with co-creation & contribution from
Deva Munay

Publisher: Inkwater Press | www.inkwaterpress.com

Paperback
ISBN-13 978-1-59299-830-2 | ISBN-10 1-59299-830-5

Printed in the U.S.A.
All paper is acid free and meets all ANSI standards for archival quality paper.

3 5 7 9 10 8 6 4 2

Dedication:
To Rhea Madrone,
Xavier Milagro and
Grace Storm, to
all of our children
you are the seed, the
sprout, the new story.
May you be nourished,
may you thrive...
in love.

Acknowledgement

Thank you, bless you, thank you to the Vestnys family for their material and spiritual support of this project. I love you all.

Deep gratitude to the incredible Moonifest Foundation (moonifest.org) whose grant subsidized the scanning and formatting of this text by the kind folks at TIS Technical Imaging Systems. TIS gently guided me through the final throes pre-publication and I am ever in their debt.

A shout out to the great presence of Inkwater Press. Your geniality and commitment to excellence makes me want to do this again.

Thank you, thank you, dear friends, family, teachers and guides. What you have given me is in these pages. I bow before you, humble, full of love. Special thanks to Eric, Xavier, Grace and Rhea for your patience and inspiration.

And to my students everywhere, each one. This book would not exist without you. All gratitude. All joy.

A note on style: This book was not written in the order it appears here. My process was organic and full of discovery. Everything transformed in the year I spent writing — the pens, the paper. My text improved. My art improved. As a result you will find inconsistencies. I am resisting the urge — right now! — to rewrite the early pages. If I can allow this expression to be artful and human — full of heart and, yes, error — perhaps I can inspire others to abandon perfection.   Create. Make. Love it all.

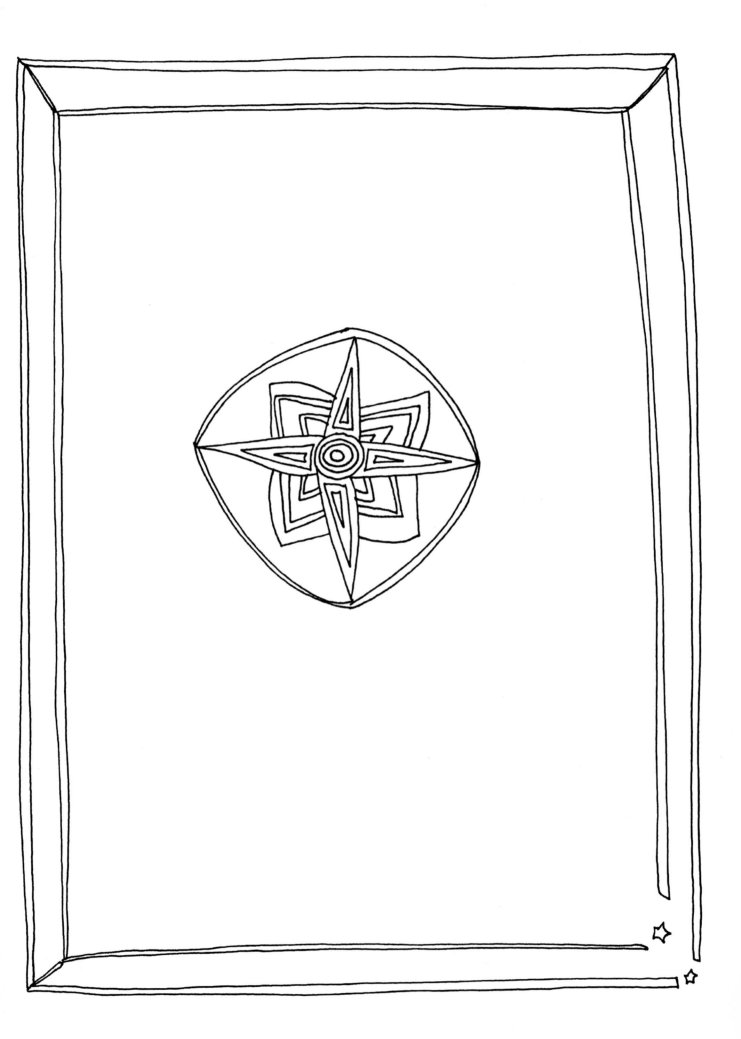

CONTENTS

Intro Pages:

Part One: Love Your Body:

CONTENTS

Part Two: Love Your Story

Part Three: Love Your Life

End Notes

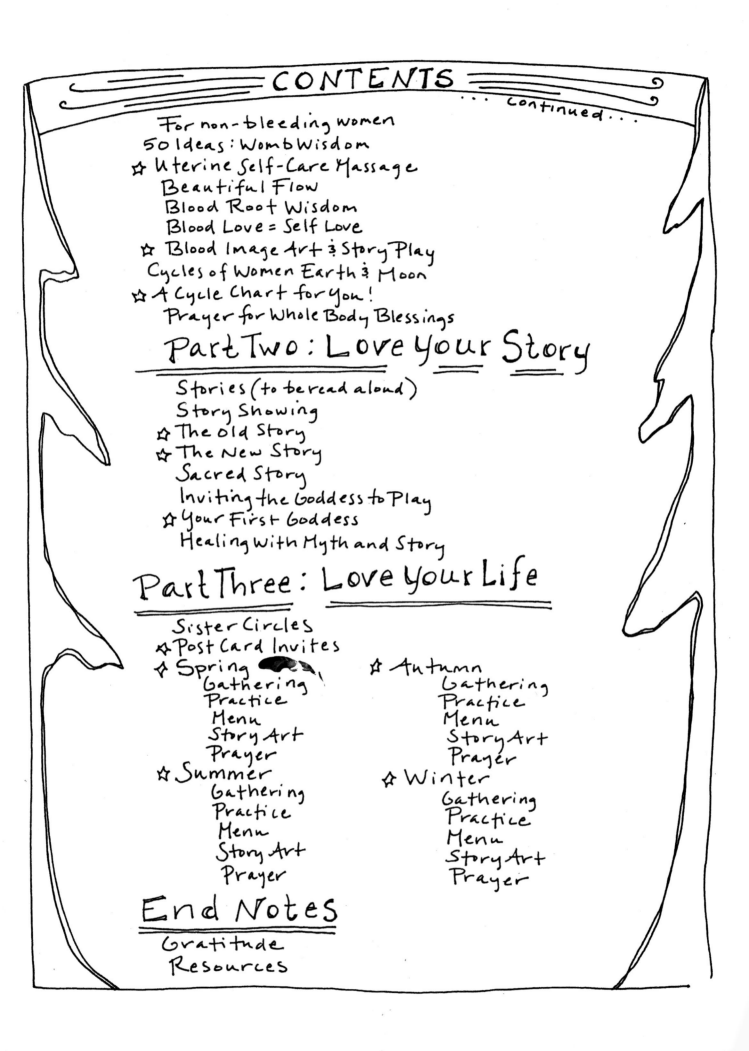

Intro Pages and Suggestions...

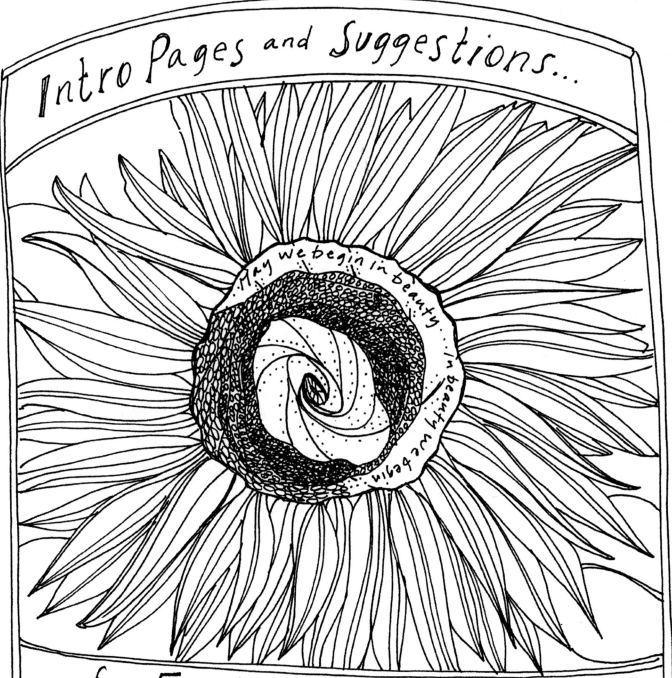

May we begin in beauty... in beauty we begin

... for Exploration...

No page numbers = freedom. This book is meant to be investigated intuitively. From front to back, end to beginning, via random section, all options are open. Your unique path is a seed, full of potential. And, as the poet Muriel Rukeyser wrote:
"The blessing is in the seed."

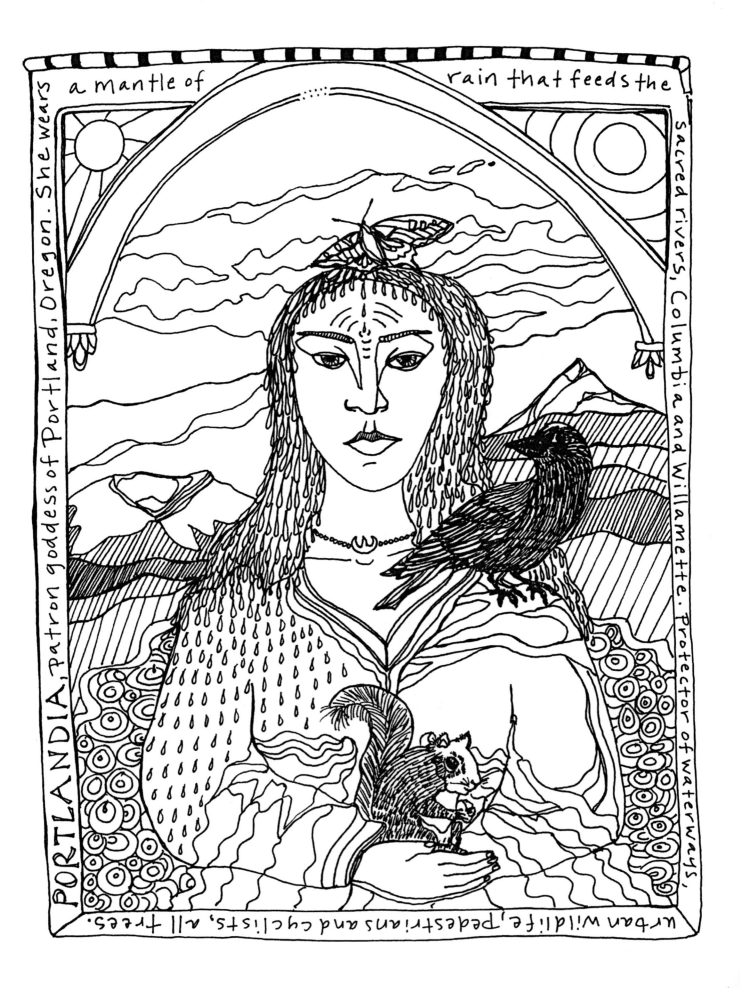

a mantle of rain that feeds the sacred rivers, Columbia and Willamette. Protector of waterways, urban wildlife, pedestrians and cyclists, all trees. PORTLANDIA, patron goddess of Portland, Oregon. She wears

Who is in transition?

The following are common states of transitional life movement:

- birth of a child
- death of a loved one
- changing occupations
- completing school
- marriage-partnering
- divorce-unpartnering
- entering new education or training
- being laid off or fired
- retiring
- children leaving home
- menarche
- menopause
- pregnancy
- moving residences
- recovery from illness or addiction
- release from incarceration or commitment
- spiritual/political/social or artistic awakening
- end of life

Life is transition, and transitions are powerful times, true opportunities for absolute transformation.

However, transitions may also be painful, chaotic, disorienting and isolating. American culture lacks the ritual solidity to bolster and fortify those in transitory life experiences. Many times, transition may cause alienation from our previous circles and communities - at least for a while. But these liminal, in-between periods can offer insight and tremendous growth if we develop the tools to ground us, to build a foundation of self-love, self-care, positive storytelling and rich daily living.

This book is dedicated to providing tools for support of vibrant and transformative transitions for all women.

What are the Tools for Transformative Transitions?

This book is a guide, a roadmap with three —must see— attractions (or sections):

☆ Love Your Body
☆ Love Your Story
☆ Love your Life

Each section offers thorough instruction in practices and experiential activities to ground and heal, to open and enliven, so that the reader may create rhythms and moments of pleasure to nourish themselves in times of trial. There are to each section corresponding ideas of connectivity & creating webs of support, of regular practice and spiritual opportunity, of attunement with nature that offer extra support.

...But I'm not in transition — can I still use the book?...

YES!! The more proactive we can be in crafting habits and practices that serve and support our highest vision for our life's purpose, the more readily we can navigate those times of inevitable transition. When we are grounded & centered and telling stories that belong to our best self, we create a reality to return to when the going gets interesting. The practices in this book are meant for affirmation and conditioning most women we know need: that you are beautiful, unique and capable of anything. That your life is a miracle!

(and it is up to you to use your miracle well...)

Entry Notes

a few thoughts on <u>knowledge</u>, <u>sex</u> and <u>fear</u>...

♡

    I once heard the poet Pattiann Rogers say, "I'm not an expert on anything." This quote has risen in the inception and crafting of this book. Deva and I began Moon Divas not because of our expertise, but to answer our soul's longing. We teach what we most need to learn: when we gather with love for our bodies, our stories and infuse our lives with the practice of that love -which is self-care- we transform the world.

    Each of you has access to the powerful knowledge of women through time, the natural world and all divinity. It does not need to be given to you. There is no product or purchase necessary. It is already in you, the wonder <u>you</u> are.

This
book
is...

... a guide to practices and
traditions we have found helpful in
the journey, this journey, toward wholeness
and joy. Some are created, some are widely
used the world over. All are intended to be
interpreted, absorbed, rebirthed and redesigned.
You will know what works for you, what challenges
you. Your body, your spirit, your heart, all
know what you need right now. Our great
work is to listen and align with inner truth.

It can be hard to trust our deep knowing
in a noisy world, especially if that trust is
blocked by fear. Fear has many purposes,
some of which protect us. But self-doubt
never aids us. Self-doubt or fear of the self,
our dreams and aspirations, our bodies, their
natural functions and eventual mortality,
these fears only serve entities that keep us
from our power. As women we are captured
by a culture of self-fear and doubt at an
early age. There are many social structures
that benefit from our disempowerment, many
industries that profit from our sorrow, pain and
constant desire to be other than we are. They do
not deserve the potent resource of our time
and attention. There are lovelier paths to take.

"Where there's fear, there's power." So goes the saying, but the power is not one of "over" but one of "within." In confronting and naming our fears, in moving toward our discomfort in order to understand its source, we achieve the strength and confidence to face another. When we avoid our fears or press them into the shadows, we negate aspects of self, spirit and psyche. We begin to fracture. Fears and limits grow in silence.

As you use this book, pay attention to your aversion. If you feel fear or anxiety, you are being challenged to look closer, not move away. The following exercise can be helpful in determining the source of your emotions. Bringing our fears to the light, with words and on paper, is the beginning of an integration.

Trust your process. Be gentle and firm with yourself. You are supported and loved. All of history is suspended by our fear. As women we must have courage.

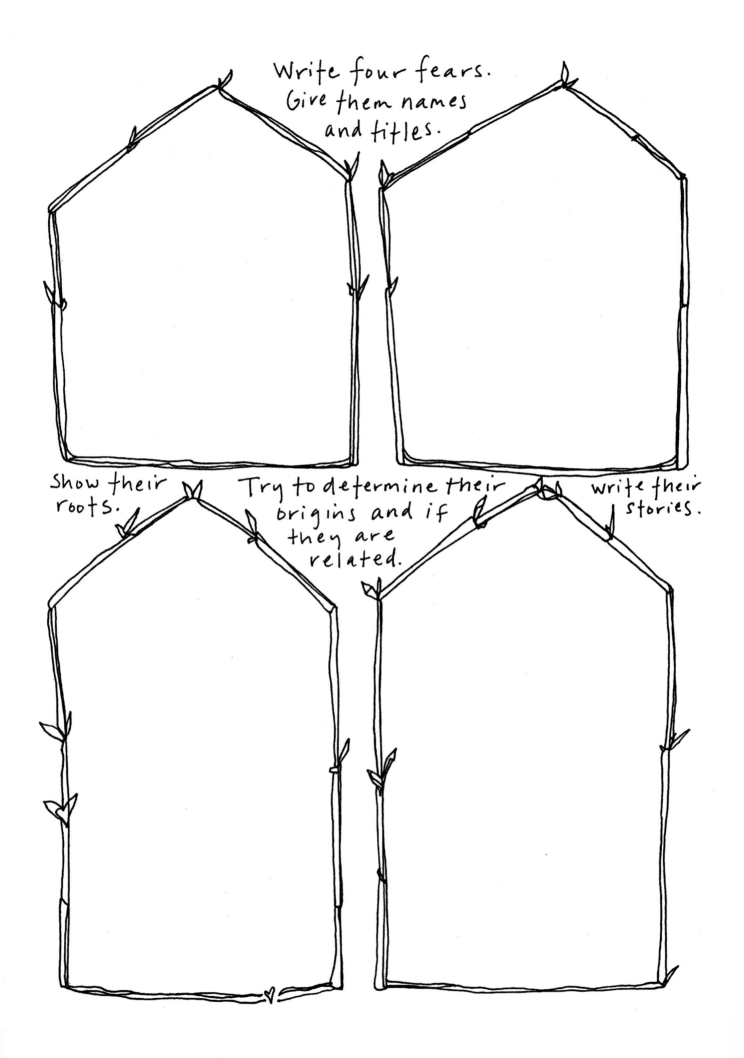

Write four fears.
Give them names
and titles.

Show their
roots.

Try to determine their
origins and if
they are
related.

write their
stories.

What does your life look like without fear?

Draw, paint, write, collage your vision here. Feel it.

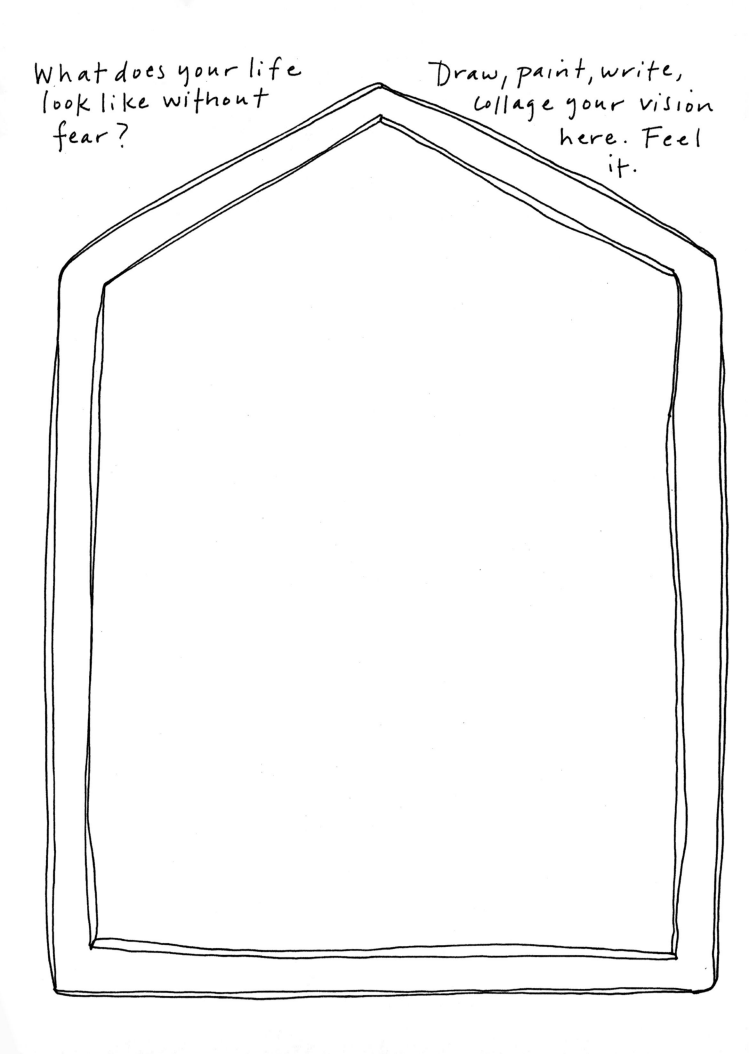

In many of us, fear and sex go hand in hand. The roots of sex-fear, body-fear, intimacy-fear, fear of rejection, are entwined and culturally our storytelling (think movies and mass media) fails us all.

Moon Divas are pro sex. But only sex without fear. Sex need not be intercourse or even partnered. Sex is our sensuality, creativity, our relation to desire and even spirit. Sex is beautiful and healing, an incredible force for transformation and fun.

We believe that when women love themselves wholly, they are able to make positive and healthy decisions about their sexual needs and expression. This is not a sex book, per se, but a book of integration, exploration and education we hope all women will come to <u>before</u> (or, at least, along with) a nourishing and vital sexual relationship with another.

...we have included an extensive list in the References section of excellent sex books for your further edification...

The place of pleasure and passage, the incredible yoni, is not forgotten in this text. Steams and baths, herbs to tone and soothe, all are mentioned. But there are many excellent texts that love the vagina in comprehensive ways, it felt neglegent to not direct a student of her body their way. Please, check them out. Tami Kent's Wild Feminine, Christiane Northrup, M.D.'s Women's Bodies, Women's Wisdom, Eve Ensler's The Vagina Monologues, Inga Muscio's Cunt, and many books on child bearing, Ina May Gaskin's Spiritual Midwifery and Susun Weed's Herbal for the Childbearing Year, celebrate and teach about our amazing yoni.

...A few months ago I had a series of sessions with Tami Kent. I realized I had never experienced before... It was non-sexual, non-clinical (think annual exam) touch in my vagina before. I realized vagina was so healing:

The Power of "Daily Practice"

What have you practiced in your life?
Widen your lens, the list is possibly large.
Writing, art, yoga, music, running, working.
Sometimes we think of practice as repetition
of an action, working to "be better" or "improve,"
but true practice from a spiritual - or even
metaphorical - point of view is bound with
intention. When we infuse any action with
our soulful intention to be present with
that action, anything may be practice. And
as you practice anything with an intention
of presence, you may also be practicing
gratitude, joy, wonder, any number of
important expansions in our daily
lenses.

♡ ♡ ♡

"Practice makes you ready." -Diana

"What nine months of attention does for an embryo, forty
early mornings will do for your gradually growing wholeness."
-Rumi

In yoga, a teacher once told me that the daily, regular practice of even a little yoga was better than attempting the big yoga blowout class once weekly... or monthly. Practice of self-care, self-love and new storytelling works the same way: small rituals, bits of devotional time spent in action, with intention, on a daily basis create habits, shift energy and manifest opportunities in ways that are nothing less than magic.

In the Moon Divas workshops we saw, time and again, that commitment to daily practice transformed our students in powerful ways, even over a relatively short period of time. Those whose practice grew into habit experienced dramatic shifts toward living the lives they'd dreamed. They created what they wanted by living intentionally and with gratitude for what they already had.

"The moment one definitely commits oneself providence moves too... Whatever you do or dream you can do, begin it. Boldness has genius, power and magic in it." — William Hutchinson Murray

Practice isn't easy. It is work, and part of the challenge is making your practice a top priority. When you prioritize your practice, you prioritize yourself. And this, for many humans, is the essence of self love.

This said, practice daily need not be at the expense of others. I have three children. My daily practice—most of the time—is to get up early and do four sun salutations before my candlelit altar while the coffee water boils, then I write for twenty minutes or so. By the time I finish this little ritual, the kids are up and ready for breakfast.

Some days are harder than others. Some days I do my sun salutations on the kitchen floor and write only a sentence, a stanza, a haiku. Every little bit counts. In a practice you can stick to, you must:

. . . use what you have . . .

♡

"Do one thing every day that scares you."
—Eleanor Roosevelt

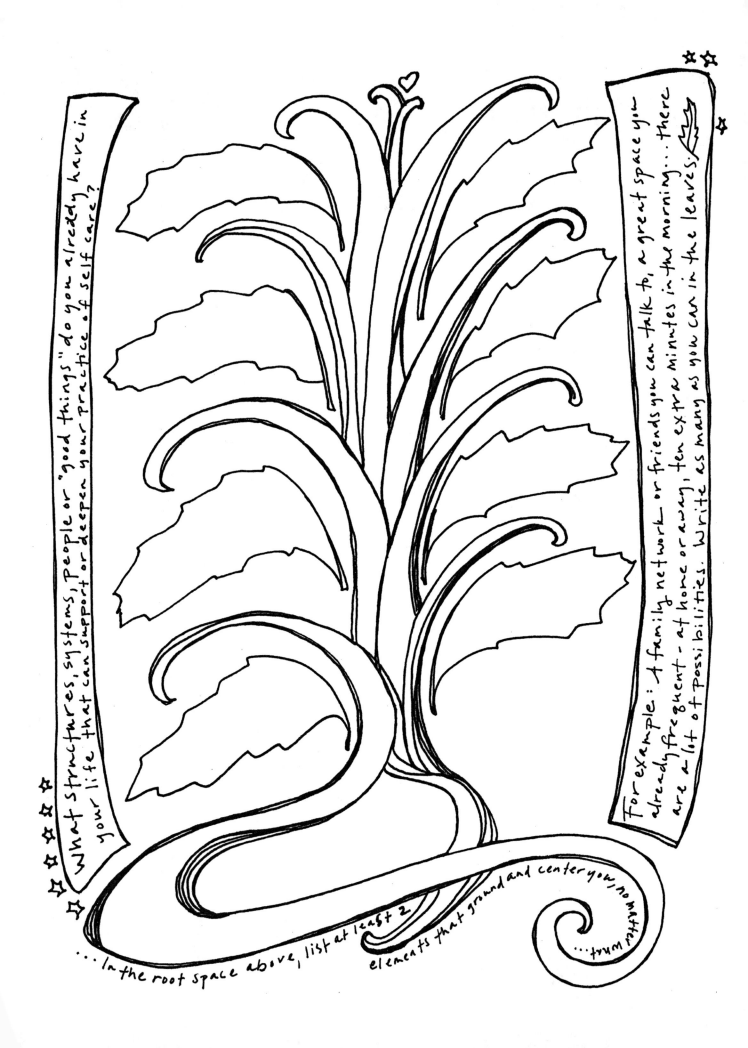

What structures, systems, people or "good things" do you already have in your life that can support or deepen your practice of self care?

For example: A family network or friends you can talk to, a great space you already frequent – at home or away, ten extra minutes in the morning…there are a lot of possibilities. Write as many as you can in the leaves.

…In the root space above, list at least 2 elements that ground and center you, no matter what…

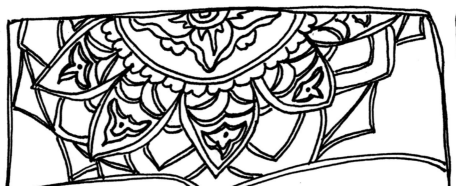

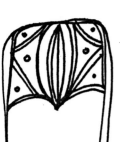

Permisson to Fail:

Because there is no failure, there are no grades for self care and loving... BUT recognizing that so many of us hold ourselves to impossible standards, and can percieve failure even when we are constantly gathering information + learning lessons to go forward a little wiser, this page gives (your name here)

_____

permission to make mistakes, large & small, forget stuff, ditch out, get dirty, make a mess, experiment and fail again and again as long as she does so with compassion... but she could fail at that too and the universe will still, in its grace, love her always.

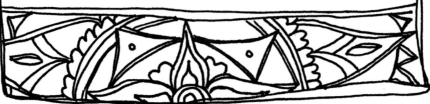

write about a time where "failure" felt good...right here...

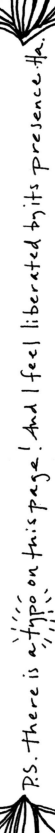

P.S. there is a typo on this page! And I feel liberated by its presence. Ha.

A Moon Divas Mantra:

There is no right way, There is only the Way

For sailing on life's storms....trial and error.... make it yours.... breathe deep · tune in · be blessed
find the rhythm.... teach to learn....love the process of changing....something big, something small, you'r mind!

Way of the wise woman.... Way of the earth.... Way of the ancestors... Way of life...

Way of the divine...Way of the universal...way of compassion... Way of connection...

Way of the ancient mother of us all........

Selfish or Self-full?

... self care keeps us caring ...

Guilt, shame and need for personal martyrdom can rise when we depend on others for our worth. Service is great, but service at the expense of health and well being hurts everyone. Often, we women may find ourselves serving out of - or with - negative emotions. In this pattern, self care may seem indulgent and we fear others criticism.

Yet when we are self-full, loving and prepared to meet whatever arrives before us, we are available to serve others with generous compassion (and good boundaries).

Awareness, in each moment, as we work and serve, can bring us to an understanding of what serves us all ....

Dandelion
"Leontodon taraxacum"

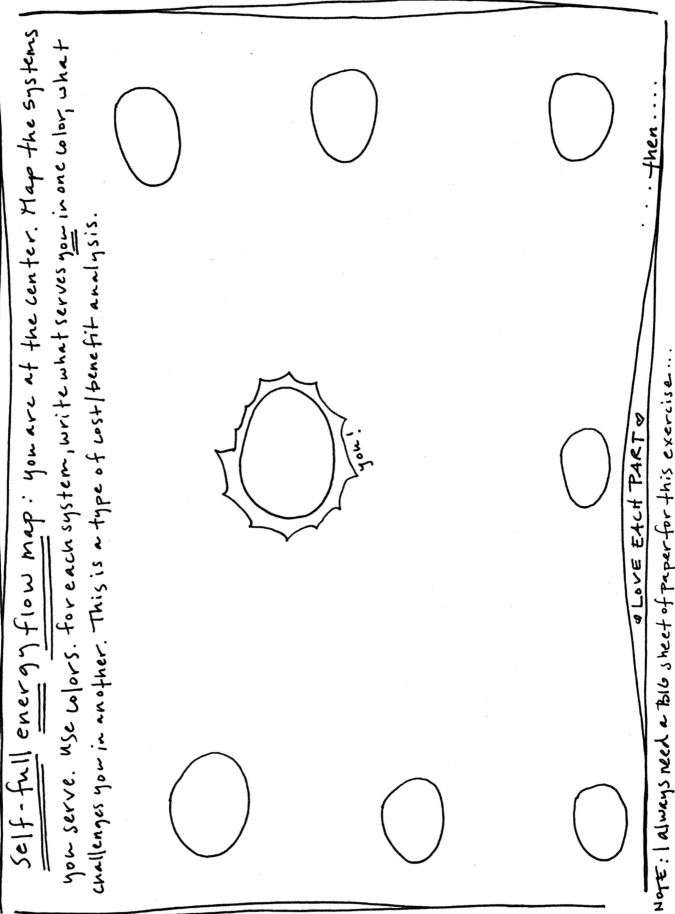

Self-full energy flow map: You are at the center. Map the systems you serve. Use colors. For each system, write what serves you in one color, what challenges you in another. This is a type of cost/benefit analysis.

you

@ LOVE EACH PART @

NOTE: I always need a BIG sheet of paper for this exercise...

...then...

We are all in transition, and loving "what is" can be an incredible challenge. Since the advent of Moon Divas I have experienced many major transitions, including single motherhood, custody negotiations, poverty, health issues, the death of relationships and birth of new ones, moving and changing communities a number of others. I return to my energy maps to remember what I value, who I truly serve and all I am grateful for in the process of living.

· · · ♡ ♡ ♡ · · ·

How do you feel, on encountering your energy systems? How does this feeling coincide with your new story, intentions or practice?

List what works:

☆ look for any connections between the service that serves you. These are your assets. Love them.

☆ Examine the costs. Give them context. What will these look like in 10 or 20 years. What can be released? What can be transformed? Can you love this too?

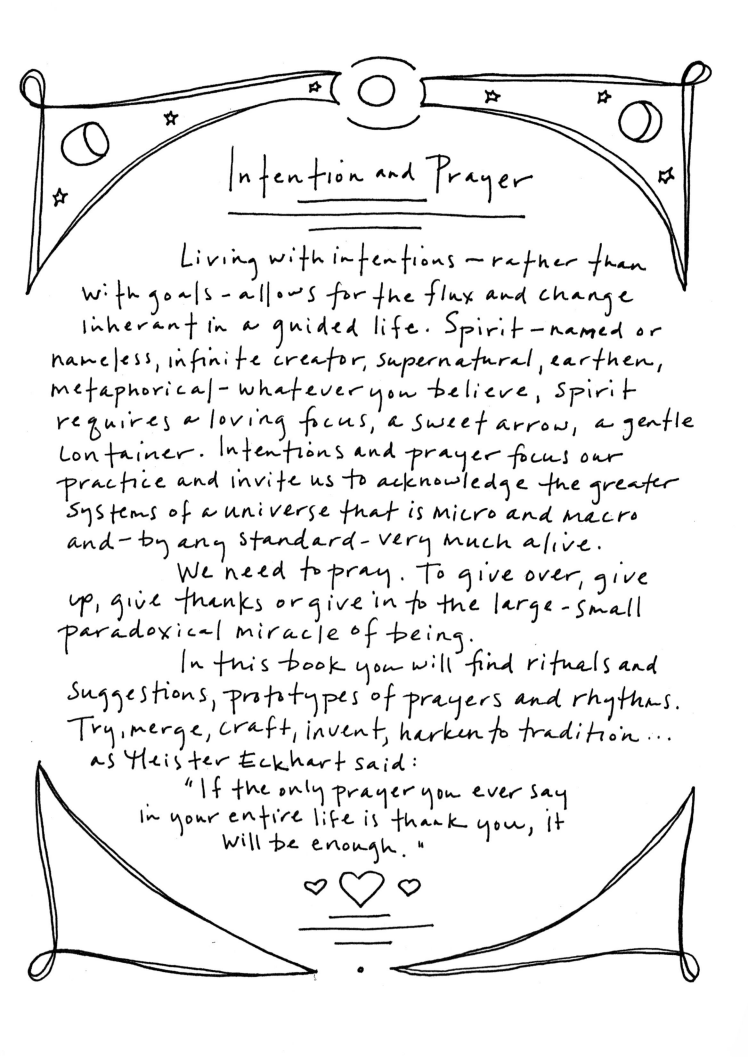

Intention and Prayer

Living with intentions — rather than with goals — allows for the flux and change inherent in a guided life. Spirit — named or nameless, infinite creator, supernatural, earthen, metaphorical — whatever you believe, spirit requires a loving focus, a sweet arrow, a gentle container. Intentions and prayer focus our practice and invite us to acknowledge the greater systems of a universe that is micro and macro and — by any standard — very much alive.

We need to pray. To give over, give up, give thanks or give in to the large-small paradoxical miracle of being.

In this book you will find rituals and suggestions, prototypes of prayers and rhythms. Try, merge, craft, invent, harken to tradition... as Meister Eckhart said:

"If the only prayer you ever say in your entire life is thank you, it will be enough."

♡ ♡ ♡

Plant your intentions! Find three seeds,
(nasturtiums and beans both work well...)
a patch of earth   outside, or in
a pot, or in   a paper cup.

Hold the seeds.   Write your
                                    intentions

1.
_____

2.
_____

3.
_____

Press the seeds into the
earth. Keep them moist
and in good light. Watch
them grow!

"Nourish
beginnings...
not all things are
blessed but the seeds
of all things are blessed.
The blessing is in the seed."
    —Muriel Rukeyser

Short term or long...

.·. Intentions may be anything, for art, life, selfcare, friendship ·.·

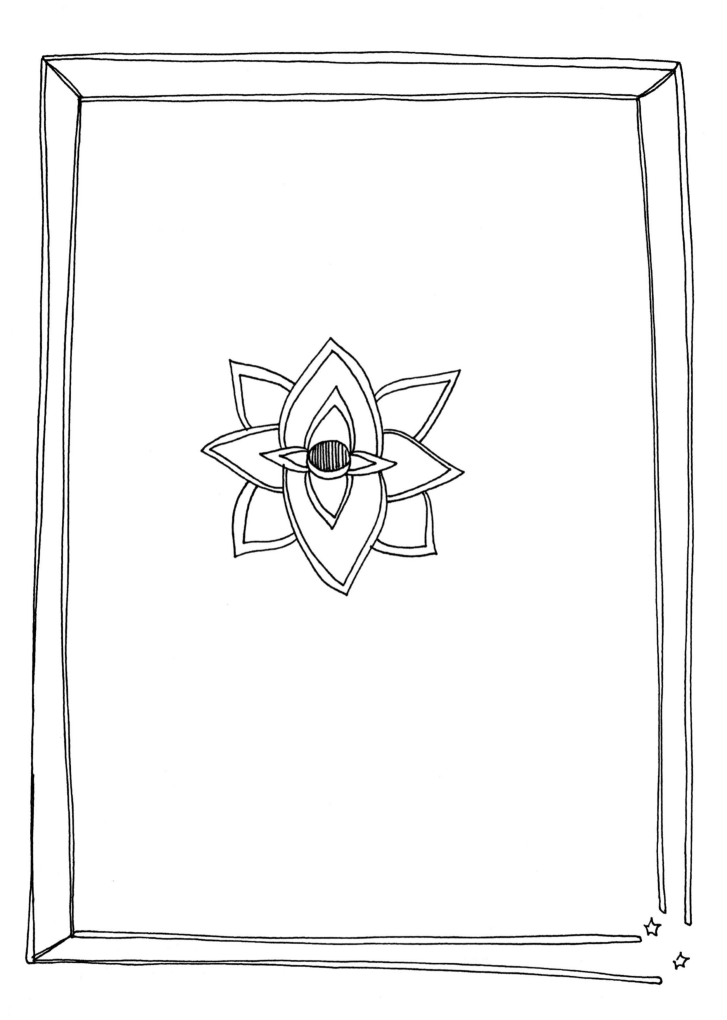

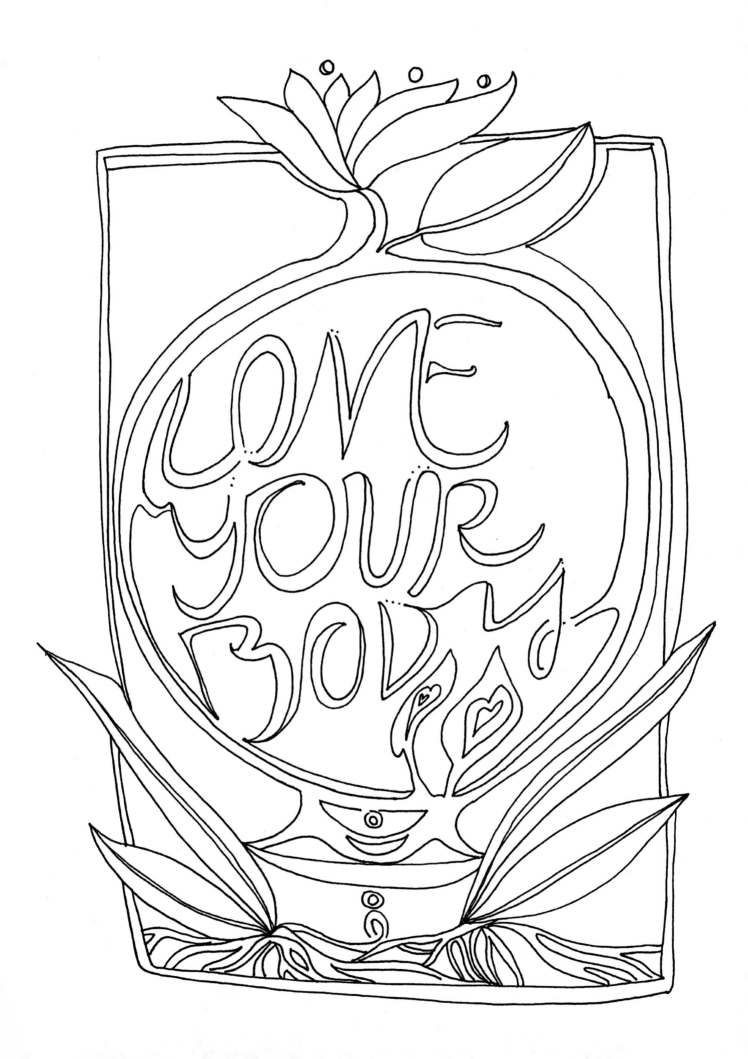

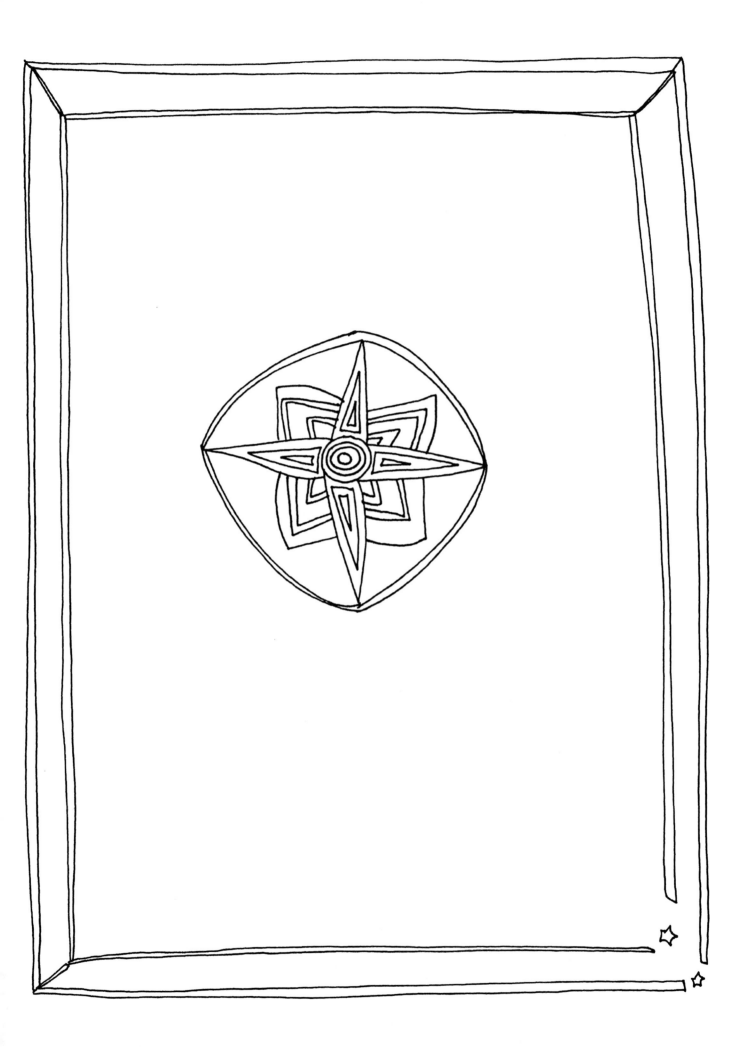

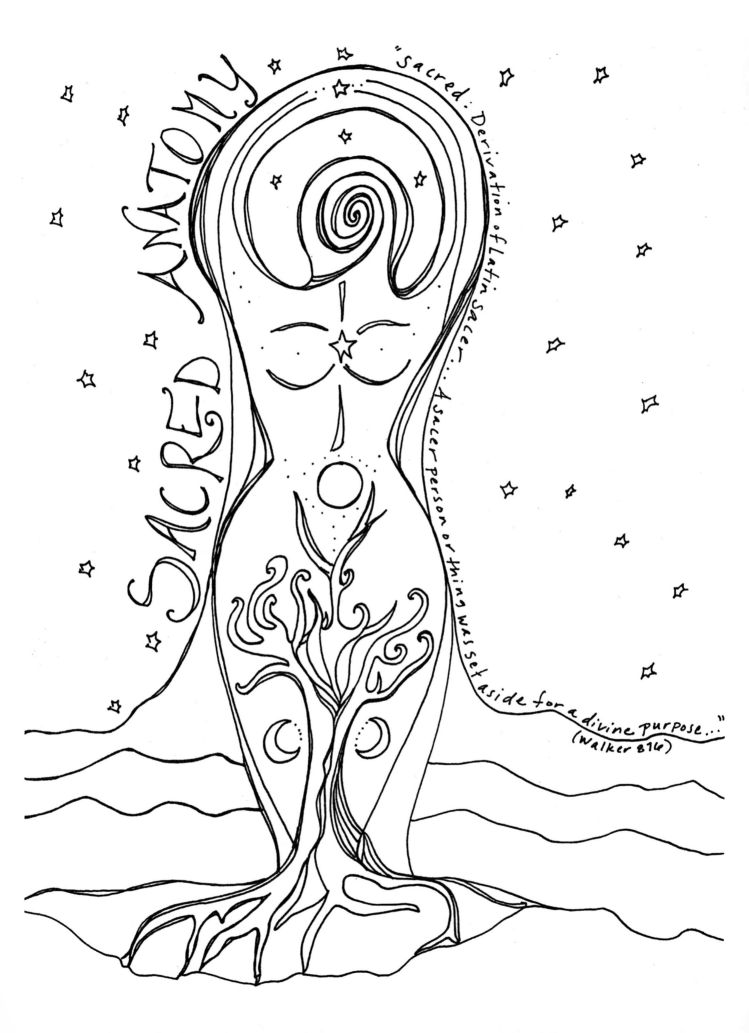

SACRED ANATOMY

"Sacred: Derivation of Latin Sacer... A sacer person or thing was set aside for a divine purpose..." (Walker 816)

What is your Sacred Anatomy?

What parts of your physical body are set aside for divine purpose?

List in the lilly's petals what you consider holy in your body, the word holy, by its pre-Christian etymology, may be defined as: "that must be preserved whole or intact, that cannot be transgressed or violated."

Holy is also connected with the old English hal: health, happiness, luck. ♥

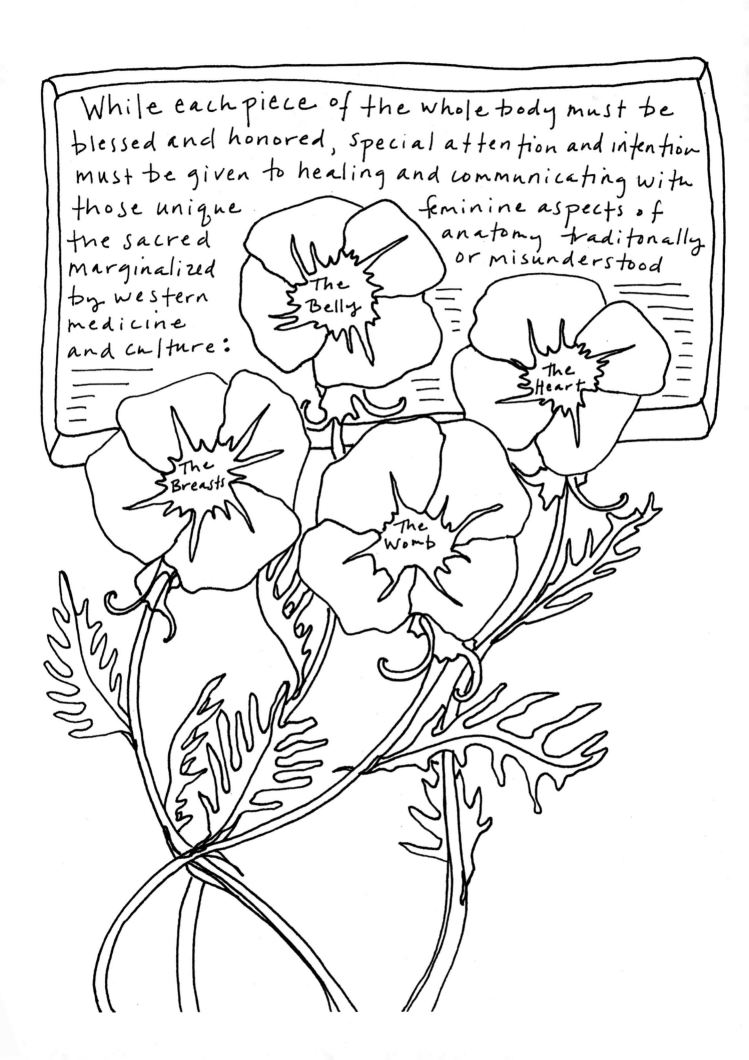

While each piece of the whole body must be blessed and honored, special attention and intention must be given to healing and communicating with those unique feminine aspects of the sacred anatomy traditonally marginalized or misunderstood by western medicine and culture:

The Belly

The Heart

The Breasts

The Womb

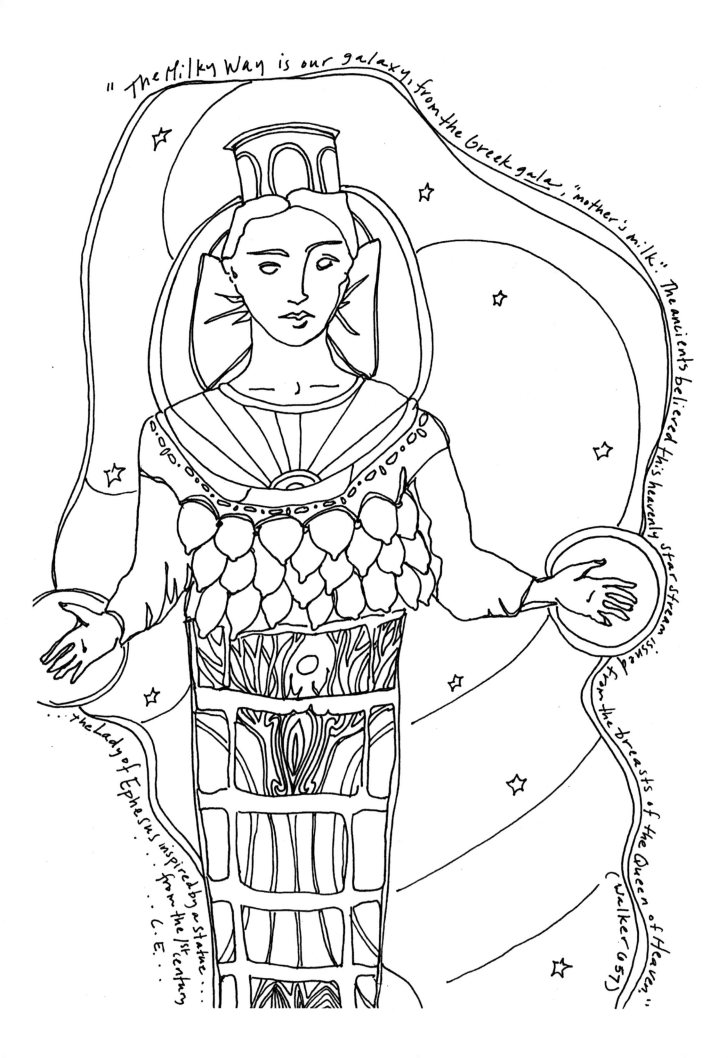

" The Milky Way is our galaxy, from the Greek gala, "mother's milk". The ancients believed this heavenly star stream issued from the breasts of the Queen of Heaven."
(Walker 657)

...the Lady of Ephesus inspired by a statue... from the 1st century ... C.E.

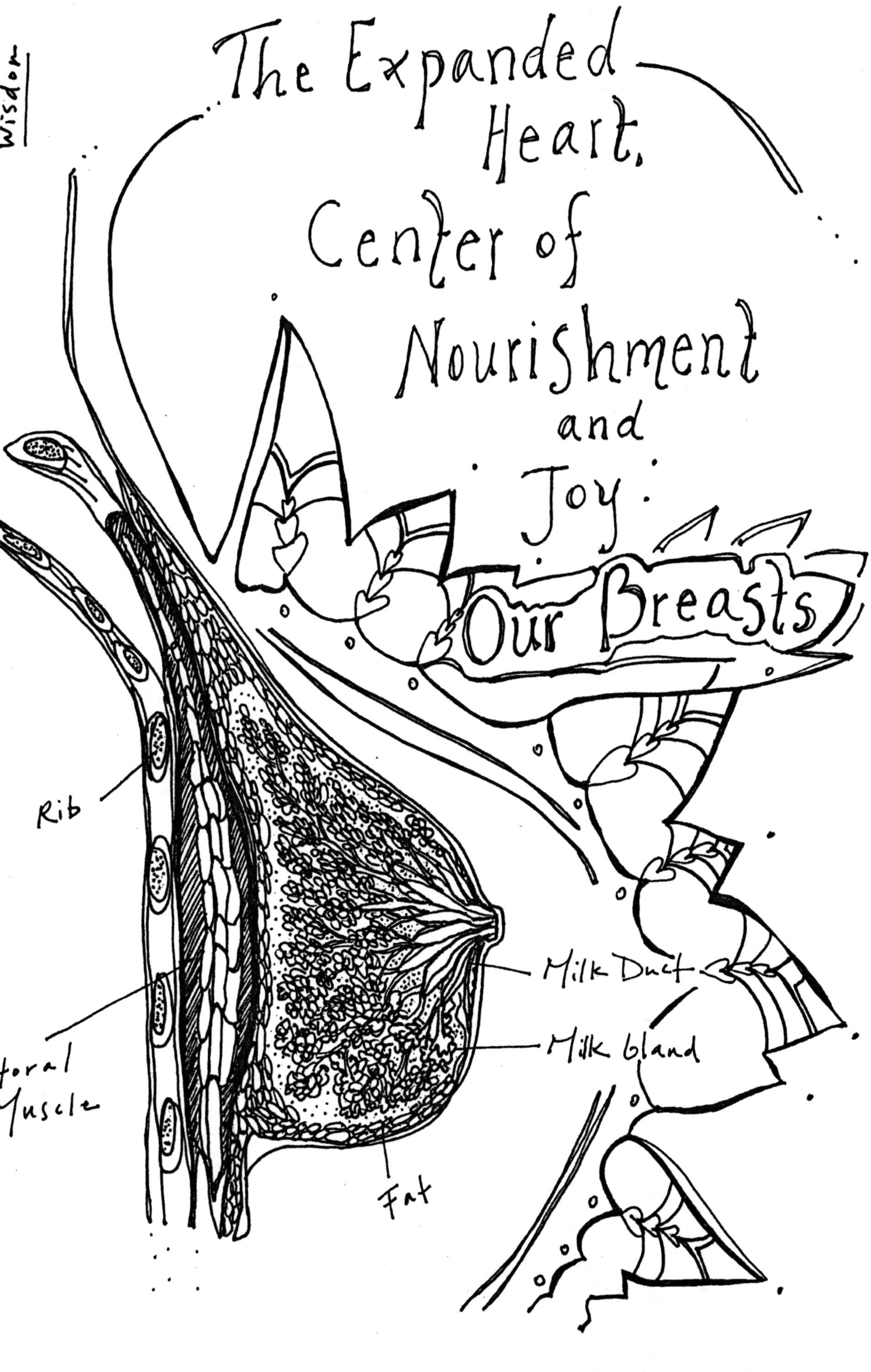

The Expanded Heart, Center of Nourishment and Joy.

Our Breasts

"The female breast is designed to provide optimal nourishment for babies and to provide sexual pleasure for the woman herself." —Dr. Christiane Northrup Woman's Bodies Woman's Wisdom

Rib

Pectoral Muscle

Milk Duct

Milk Gland

Fat

... your breasts record the journey of your feminine evolution, a winding path ...

One of the great discoveries of my early adulthood occurred one evening when I was nineteen and living away from home for the first time in a house with three other women: future Moon Divas Deva and Riley and our beloved friend Anne.

I can't remember the why, only that we for some reason gathered in the bathroom before the mirror and removed our shirts.

There stood four beautiful women with four entirely unique sets of breasts: round, large, small, pink, big nipples, little nipples. All perfectly imperfect. All our own.

I realized my perception of my own breasts was based on nothing real. Rarely had I seen the breasts of other women who weren't models or actors. In front of that mirror — the mirror of other living, breathing women — it became much easier to accept our individuality. To honor, appreciate and laugh.

Where I had carried for so many years a sense of discomfort and shame about my breasts, after that night I found only ease and peace.

Breast Affirmation #1: I am whole, healthy, supported and loved.

Since that night of mirroring nearly twenty years ago I have experienced many things that have changed my breasts and my relationship to them: travel to countries where breasts are not taboo, years of pregnancy and breastfeeding infants and toddlers, a lover who adored my breasts and awakened me to their erotic potential, a breast lump diagnostic process, breast self-care massage and teaching breast love to women of all ages. My breasts, older, wizened, more beautiful and precious to me than ever, hold stories.

All breasts carry stories. Some of the most incredible healing I've witnessed transpired in circles of women who told those stories. Circles of women who later bathed each other in a flower bath ritual, honoring and celebrating our holy beauty together.

○ What is your breast story?
○ Write the first one that comes to mind, without censorship, on the following page. It may be funny, sexy, joyful or painful. By sharing our stories we make it possible to claim our bodies for our own.

Breast Affirmation #2:
I give and receive in ease and gratitude.

Write your breast story here. See what they hold.

Keep your hand moving as you write.

Breast Affirmation #3:

I adapt with fluidity to life's changes.

~BREAST LOVE ~ DAY~

♡ ANY DAY ♡ EVERY DAY ♡

MAY BE CELEBRATED ALONE OR WITH FRIENDS!

♡ To prepare for breast love day, make an infused oil or/and tea infusion and prepare your favorite foods in advance. Clear the schedule, mark the calendar. Be excited!

♡ Choose three activities from the Breast Love sheet on the next page and become giddy with excitement! Oh. I said that already...

♡ Set your dream space. Hold your breasts as you fall asleep and bless them.

♡ Wake <u>slowly</u>, as peacefully as possible. Breathe into your breasts and heart. Gently massage your breasts and the surrounding area above them, beneath your arms to stimulate the lymph glands.

♡ Keep a slow and easeful place through the day for reflection and awareness. How do your breasts experience the world? What is comfortable or uncomfortable for them? Strive for moments of high pleasure and boundary stretching. Give yourself love.

Breast Affirmation #4:
I center in my holy heart with gratitude and love.

♡ Breast Love Squares ♡

- Find a breast image from history or art you love and frame it.
- Learn your breasts. Visit them daily and mind map their topography.
- Treat your chest and breasts to the same bathing, skin care and treatment as your face.
- Wear a shirt or dress that shows a little "too much". Why is it too much?
- Write a breast haiku.

- Take your breasts to the movies. Ask for a review.
- Find pleasure in your breasts, just as they are.
- Take a picture of your breasts. Show them as they are — Love them.
- Go skinny dipping or visit a sauna or hot spring.
- Ask a woman to tell her breast story.

- Hug yourself. Be firm. Hug again...
- Practice affirming touch: examine your breasts with positive thoughts.
- Make sure your bra is comfortable and fits properly. Then make it beautiful.
- Sunshine and fresh air feel great on the breast. Be free!
- Experiment with fabrics. What feels good close to your bare breasts?

- Meditate on the fact that the whole of humanity — until the 1950's — was nursed at the breast of a woman.
- Check out the book: "The Family of Women" beautiful photographs!
- Support a nursing mother with a kind gesture.
- Teach someone a breast positive fact, such as:
- Make breast prints. Revel in their shape.

- Scent your breasts with your favorite natural oil.
- Use body paint to decorate your breasts. What images do they carry?
- Move! Breasts need free motion on occasion. Lose the bra...
- Indulge in a castor oil pack on your breasts.

♡ INFUSED BREAST OIL ♡

...for massage...

you need:
- 1 jar with a tight lid - DRY
- organic almond or olive oil

stuff the jar with the fresh or wild-harvested herbs of your choice. On a Moon Divas herb walk we used:
- pine
- yarrow
- yellowdock

but many aromatic or culinary herbs such as rosemary, oregano thyme, chamomile, dandelion blooms, & rose - can be used and are healing. Herb books are useful, as is a cultivated intuition. Ask the plants and your body what is needed.

Completley cover fresh herbs with oil (make sure your herbs don't have water or dew on them). Let sit in a warm spot with light for a few weeks. Strain and use!

Information from Deva Munay, LMT

♡ BREAST TEA and BATH ♡

Warmth stimulates and soothes... water nourishes and replenishes. In and on the body, warm water is alchemy. Add plant friends from the garden and you have magic.

Mineral rich herbs such as Raspberry Leaf, Nettle and Red Clover support and tone the body's tissues and systems. What grows near you? Find a plant you enjoy and work to learn from it, play with it. Plant relationships feed the soul.

For bathing, the addition of your favorite plant friend, harvested with love, and aromatic petals - fresh or dried - to a hot bath is a drink of restoration for the whole body.

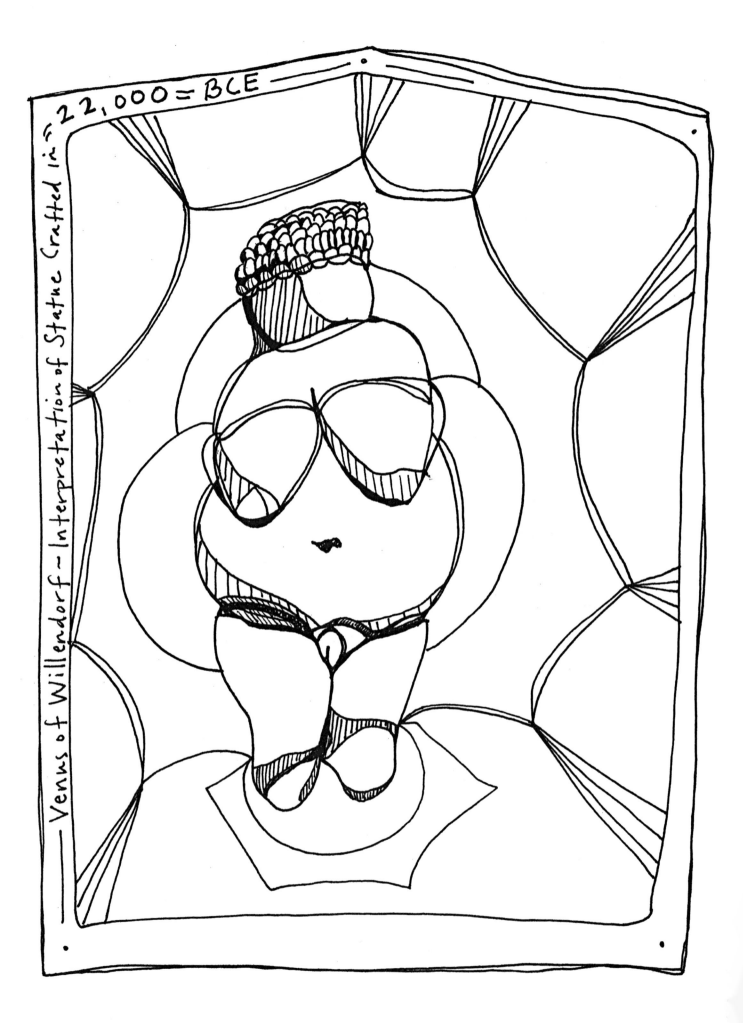

— 22,000 = BCE —

Venus of Willendorf ~ Interpretation of Statue Crafted in

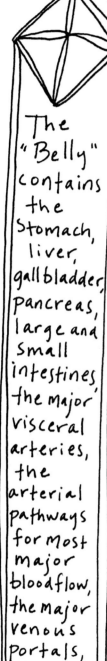

The "Belly" contains the stomach, liver, gallbladder, pancreas, large and small intestines, the major visceral arteries, the arterial pathways for most major bloodflow, the major venous portals, the kidneys and adrenal glands.

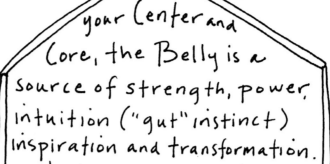

your Center and Core, the Belly is a source of strength, power, intuition ("gut" instinct) inspiration and transformation.

In the energetic image of the chakra system the Belly is a yellow gold. The Sanskrit word for this third chakra, located above your navel at your solar plexus (a term whose roots mean "network of the sun" and refer to the complex of nerves located there), is "Manipura." This translates to "city of gems."

A place of heat, light, physical and spiritual importance, the Belly is also the location of much enmity and dissatisfaction. It is a place we are prone to covering and hiding, a place where we may store unexpressed anger or feed grief. To embrace the Belly we must reveal true hunger and find ways to nourish ourselves.

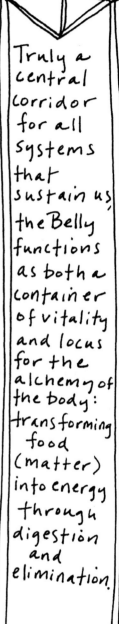

Truly a central corridor for all systems that sustain us, the Belly functions as both a container of vitality and locus for the alchemy of the body: transforming food (matter) into energy through digestion and elimination.

PHYSICALLY	MENTALLY
energy · vitality · strength	will · insight · transmutation

Building and growing a relationship with the Belly begins
with a multi-leveled question:

What are you Hungry for?

EMOTIONALLY	SPIRITUALLY
trust · self-worth · risk	creativity · inspiration · joy

It is the place many of us would rather skip, this soft spot, this tender middle with its folds and marks. Yet its muscles ease the spine, carry us upright, forward and alive. Our Belly hunger is not for thin or flat: those are recent aesthetics, rooted in stories that belong to so few. What about power? Strength, solidity, stamina? How does the story change when we strive to be strong versus thin? How many ways are there to be thin? How many ways are there to be strong?

What is your belly story? Write one on the following page. Look for clues when you are done. When do you serve your belly, your center, what it needs to feel satisfied?

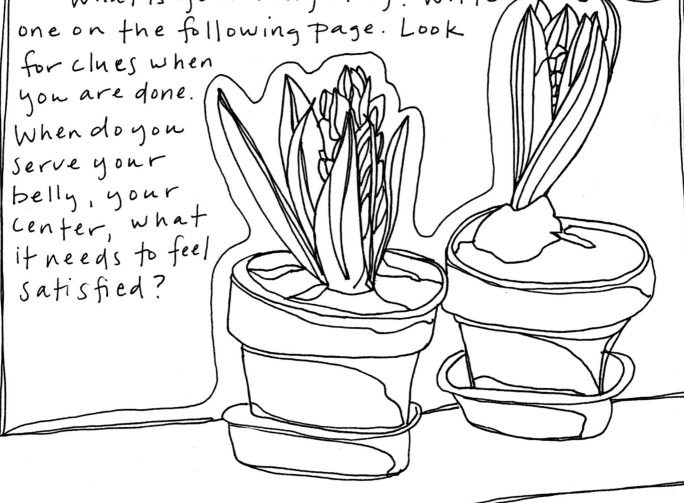

WRITE YOUR BELLY STORY....

After, spend some time with your hand on
your belly. Breathe into that core.

• GRATITUDE • ABUNDANCE • FOOD •
What are We Digesting?

In planning the Moon Divas workshops Deva and I realized that food, eating and being fed, were essential parts of the self-care experience. For many women, ourselves included, food means work, time, and can trigger issues of lack, guilt and servitude - to name a few. We decided to cook locally grown organic produce into seasonal whole foods meals for our participants. The process, from purchasing the ingredients to crafting the meals, to sitting down together and savoring, slowly, together the meal was amazing.

Meals became more communal as workshop students participated in work trade: five or six women arriving early and contributing their unique skills made the preparation so easy and the outcome more delicious. We began telling stories at meals, offering gratitude for all before us. We began walking after meals, holding our bellies with loving hands. We realized Elizabeth Gilbert was onto something: you must Eat first, then Pray, and Love.

♥ BELLY · LOVE ♥

A Blessing (invented when my children were small):

To the earth that gives us this food, To the Sun that helps it to grow, To the People who tend it and harvest it, And to the creator who is all we give our thanks. ♥

(Then we would go round the table and each would say one thing we were grateful for and one thing we wish)...

♥ Prepare food together with family or friends... Share with neighbors or take a class. Begin the experience of sharing food in community.

♥ Be kind to your sources. Seasonal local food nourishes body and the extended systems we require for survival. Find out where your food comes from and imagine a way to make it closer.

♥ Mealtime is a sacred act. When we pause for a moment to give thanks to all that synthesis on our plate (earth, air, the sun, water, people, creatures) we change the meaning of the food and our relationship to it. Our digestive processes begin with our thoughts. Gratitude is a potent start to any meal.

♥ Eat what makes you feel amazing. Not just in the moment, but in the whole entire day.

A Blessing (adapted from a Unitarian prayer):

The food we are about to eat Is earth, air, water and sun, Compounded through the alchemy of many plants. It is also the result of the labors of many beings and creatures, and we are grateful for it. May it give us strength, health and joy, And may it increase our love.

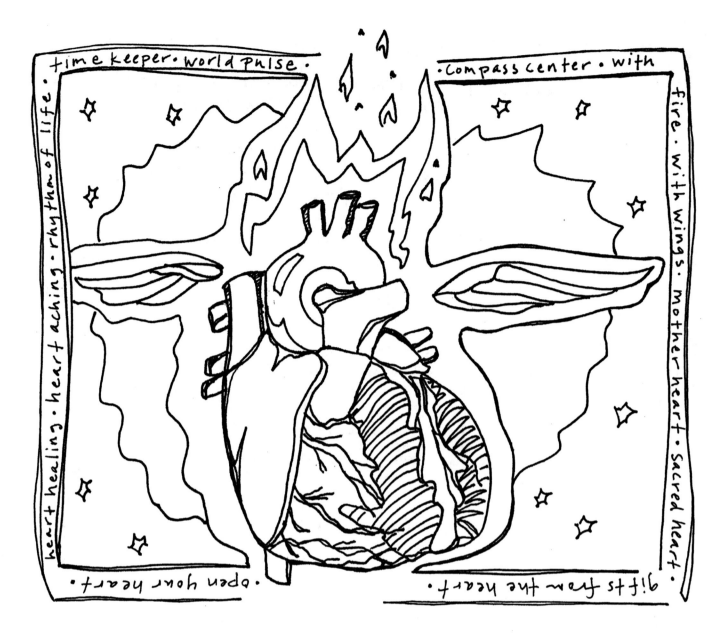

time keeper · world pulse · ·compass center · with fire · with wings · mother heart · sacred heart · gifts from the heart · open your heart · heart healing · heart aching · rhythm of life

Our Heart

"We are at the threshold. We are going to see change. If we can create the vision in our heart, it will spread. As women of wisdom, we cannot be divided. As bringers of light, we have no choice but to join together."
— Agnes Baker Pilgrim —

At four weeks after your mother's egg and father's sperm merged, your tiny, rudimentary heart began to beat.

At eight weeks, when you were an inch long, your perfect heart was fully formed and dancing inside you. It beats 100,000 times each day.

"_Ab_ was the Egyptian word for "heart-soul," most important of the seven souls bestowed by the seven birth-goddesses... The _ab_ was most important because it was the central blood-soul emanating from the essence of the mother... the Egyptian hieroglyphic sign for _ab_ was a dancing figure and as a verb it meant "to dance." This referred to the mystic dance of life going on inside the body - the heartbeat... So vital was the idea of the heartbeat in Oriental religions that the very center of the universe was placed "within the heart" by Tantric sages... Jesus' divinity was "the moon dwelling in the heart." His Sacred Heart was described as... "the temple in which dwells the life of the world," as a rose, a cup, a treasure, a spring, as the furnace of divine love... as a bridal chamber." "

(Walker 375-377)

Locate your heart. It sits in the center of your chest between the lungs, the bottom tipped slightly to the left. It is about the size of your two fists together. The aorta, the largest artery, is the size of a garden hose. The capillaries, the smallest blood vessels, can fit ten inside the width of a human hair.

Breathe into the rhythm of your heart. Right now it is circulating the five to six quarts of blood in your body two to three times every minute. In one day your blood travels a distance of 12,000 miles.

Give thanks. The heart needs and deserves our love and gratitude. Today heart disease is the number one cause of death for women in the United States. We must tend, open and heal our hearts.

.: Information from Deva Munay, LMT :.

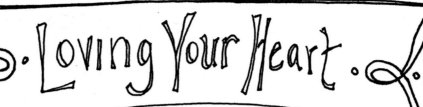
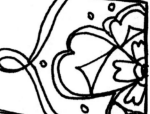

Loving Your Heart

What does it mean to live from the heart? In the space below make a list of 100 things you love. If you have a friend close by (or close by phone) share your list. How do you feel? How does your heart feel?

"The heart is the thousand-stringed instrument
That can only be tuned with Love."
— Hafiz

MORE ♥ LOVE
for your Heart

Heart Wings partner exercise: have someone you love place their hands on the back side of your heart between your shoulder blades. See your heart with wings, see them sprout from the heat of your partner's hands. Breathe them big. Describe them aloud. ♥ Then, switch partners. ♥♥ Record your heart with vision on the next page. write draw collage the wings of your sweet heart.

Rose Water for bathing and drinking: Pick 3-5 organic roses just beginning to bloom (smaller roses require more) Twist the blooms between both hands just once and place in a glass jar. Cover with water and refrigerate overnight. As you drink or bathe in the water imagine your heart blooming open.

We know stress, anxiety, worry and fear hurt our hearts. System tonics like the tea below nourish and soothe the nerves while quieting the mind. Make and drink often! ↙↘ ♥

Heart Song infusion: equal parts
- ◎ chamomile
- ◎ oat tops (oat straw)
- ◎ spearmint
- ◎ motherwort

¼-½ cup herbs (depending on desired strength) Place in a quart jar Cover with boiling water and add lid. Steep 30-60 mins. Strain & Drink. ♥

Move from your heart: dance, swim, skip, roll, tickle, race, hike, stretch, walk, run, jump, slide, spin, drum, hokey-pokey, tumble, twist, be sweaty. Be, breathing, beating in strength, in time. Move, every day. Make it fun. Move with friends. Move when you are tired, move when it is a challenge. Movement is heart love. Regular, long-term movement is essential to heart health and joy. ♥

HEART ♥ WINGS

_____ 'S PORTRAIT _____
DATE

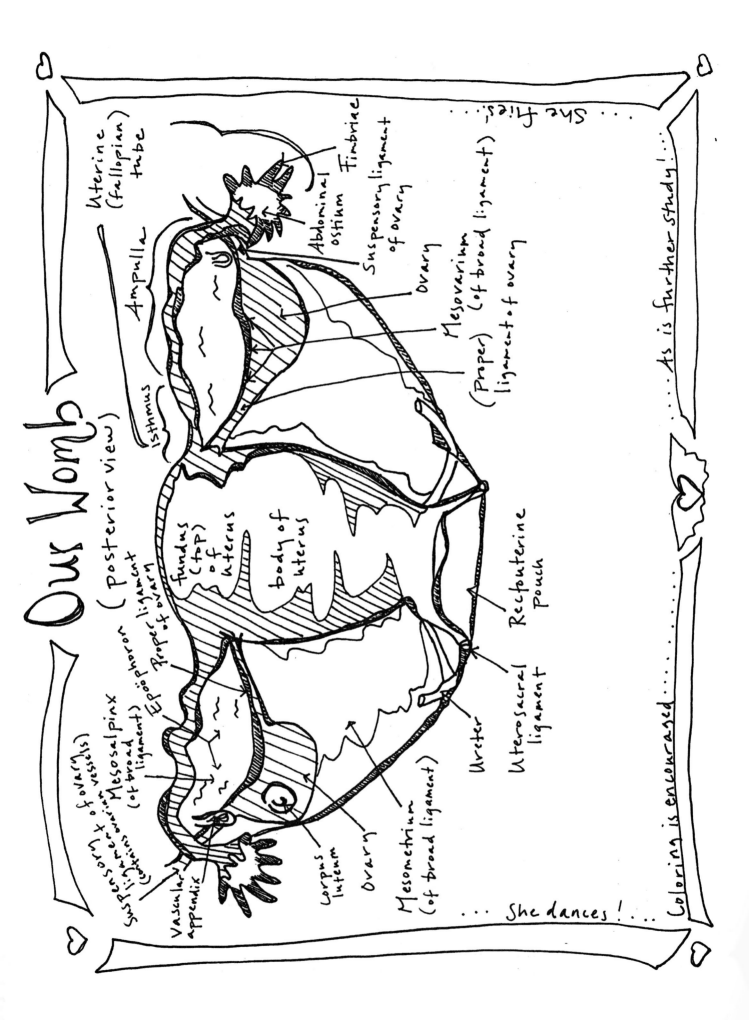

Our Womb

(posterior view)

Uterine (fallopian) tube

Ampulla

Isthmus

Abdominal ostium

Fimbriae

Suspensory ligament of ovary

Ovary

Mesovarium (of broad ligament)

(Proper) ligament of ovary

Suspensory ligament of ovary

Mesovarium

Mesosalpinx (of broad ligament)

Epoöphoron

Proper ligament of ovary

Vascular appendix

fundus (top) of uterus

body of uterus

Rectouterine Pouch

Uterosacral ligament

Ureter

Mesometrium (of broad ligament)

Ovary

Corpus luteum

She flies.....

.....As is further study!.....

.....She dances!.....

Coloring is encouraged.......

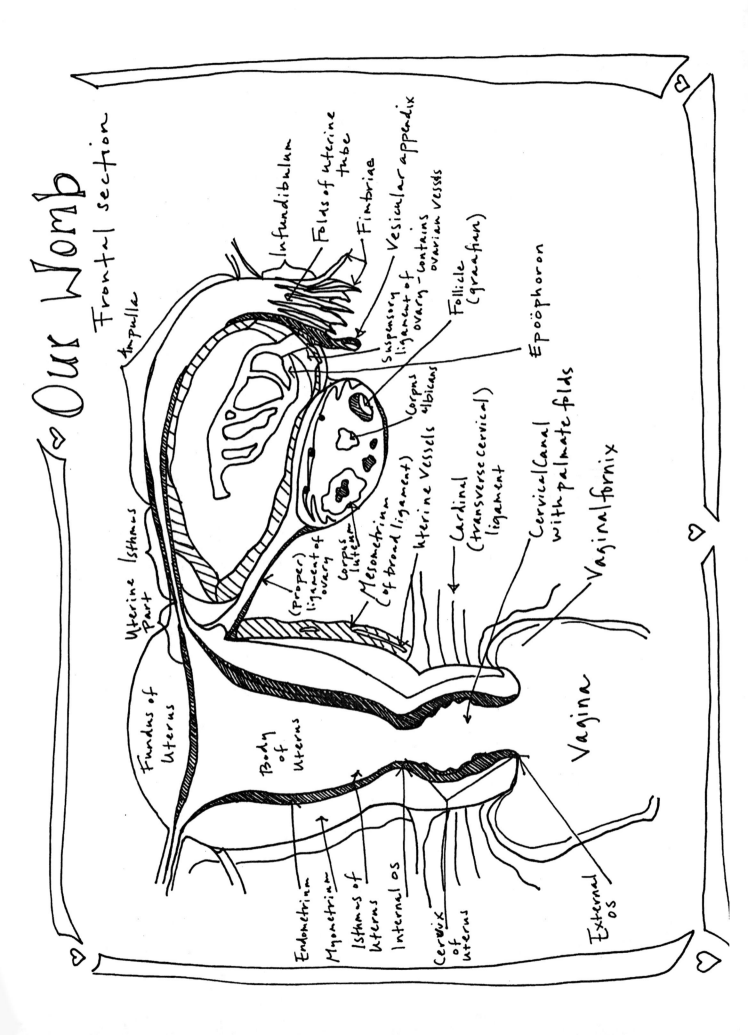

Our Womb
Frontal section

Ampulla

Uterine Isthmus Part

Fundus of Uterus

Body of Uterus

Endometrium
Myometrium
Isthmus of Uterus
Internal os

Cervix of Uterus

Infundibulum
Folds of uterine tube
Fimbriae
Vesicular appendix
Suspensory ligament of ovary — contains ovarian vessels
Follicle (graafian)

Corpus albicans
Corpus luteum
(Proper) ligament of ovary
Mesometrium (of broad ligament)
Uterine vessels
Cardinal (transverse cervical) ligament
Epoöphoron
Cervical Canal with palmate folds
Vaginal fornix

Vagina

External os

♡ Our Womb ♡

Originator and beginning place for each human on this planet, our womb is a place of timeless wisdom and incredible power. With the twin containers of the ovaries and the dancing fallopian tubes, the womb is the center where we hold our creative potential, our holy fire.

"The Sanskrit word for any temple or sanctuary was garbha-grha, "womb."

The oldest oracle in Greece... was named Delphi, from delphos, "womb".

Megalithic tombs and barrow-mounds were designed as "wombs" to give rebirth to the dead... womb-temples and womb-tombs point backward to the matriarchal age where only feminine life magic was thought efficacious."

(Walker 1091-1092)

The womb was revered for thousands of years as the source of all life, a literal and allegorical vessel of creation. Indiginous cultures worldwide still hold the womb in esteem and honor, but in the western contemporary paradigm, the womb is, at best, forgotten.

At worst, she is pathologized and her natural processes ~ menstruation, birth, menopause - villified as things to be "dealt" with. We have been sold a forgetting. We forget that the first calendar was lunar, based on a woman's rhythmic cycles. We forget that once, our blood was holy and created the world (see the ancient stories from every continent for reference here). We forget that when we love and honor our cycles and wombs, we honor every woman, every human, all life.

And there lies tremendous power.

As Moon Divas, we commit to loving our bodies. Even those places that are—for whatever reason—difficult to love. Part of loving means knowing, embracing the history and mystery of the body. Few physical organs have such a complicated story as that of the womb. What is your womb story? What about the stories of your mothers and grandmothers? When do you notice your womb? What does she look like?

Draw a portrait of your womb. It may be literal or symbolic. It may require several attempts, or be added to over time. Ask your womb to guide you.

Write a womb story here. It may be one of your own or one of your lineage. We each have many. If your womb has been removed, its essence remains. Honor its history, or write it a letter.

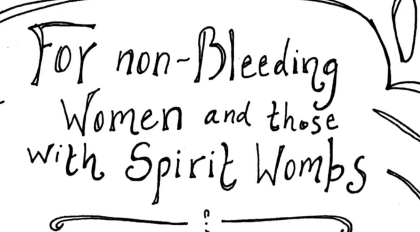

For non-Bleeding Women and those with Spirit Wombs

Womb wisdom is accessible to anyone. The pulse of the divine creatrix beats within us all. If your womb place is empty, for whatever reason, you have only to call on the spirit of the sacred feminine. Her energy is yours, for she belongs to all who seek her in themselves.

Every exercise in this book can be performed with or without a physical womb. Abdominal massage, cycle charting and moon rituals are healing for all, adhere us again to the gentle pulse of this world we love—and who loves us back.

Believe and trust. Be gentle with yourself. Appreciate and love the absolute wonder that you are!

Womb Wisdom and Self Care

50 Ways to Celebrate Your Second Heart

Take a womb day off each month. Rest, relax, connect.

Lie on the earth, the grass, the beach—the womb of all that lives.

Mentor a girl on the cusp of womanhood. Be a role model, a teacher.

Practice self-care massage regularly—get to know your inner guide.

Dance from your womb—alone or with friends!

Paint a womb picture—a portrait of or for your womb.

Ask about your birth. What is your mother's womb story?

Did anyone else share your mother's womb? What about your grandmother's? Investigate womb lineage.

Greet your womb each morning before you rise. Place your hand on her for a few breaths. Say hello.

As you set your sleep space at night, ask your womb for dreams. Write down what arrives in the morning.

Drink regular infusions of raspberry leaf tea. Rich in iron, niacin and maganese, it is a tasty womb-specific tonic. To make an infusion (Susun Weed style) add two handfuls of leaves to a quart jar. Fill with boiling water, cap and let sit four or more hours (Weed 242). Strain and drink. Delicious warm or cold!

Be a womb hystorian! Some ideas include:

Reading Womb-Positive books! Such as:

Cunt by Inga Muscio

Wild Feminine by Tami Lynn Kent

Share your favorite books!

The Red Tent by Anita Diamant

Woman and Nature by Susan Griffin

The Alphabet Versus the Goddess by Leonard Shlain

The Woman's Encyclopedia of Myths and Secrets by Barbara Walker

Record her story, your story... Write about:

Your first menstruation how did you feel? has it changed?

Your mother's first menstruation. What does she say?

Childbirth. Experiences. Hopes + fears. Witness. Human + womb history.

Menopause. Experiences. Hopes + fears. What do you know? What do you need to learn?

Write your womb a letter. Ask questions like:

What do you need from me?

What does the world need from my womb?

What are we trying to birth into being? What outlet do I need for the creation?

What is your favorite activity? Where is your favorite place?

Then, have your womb write back. Allow for the connection to flow through you. Listen deeply, this is your connection to ancestry, fertility, art and power.

Create a collage from your womb. This may be a vision board or simply an image response.

When you are faced with a decision, check in with your womb. The ceremony on the next page can be helpful.

Educate yourself about uterine orgasm. Research the womb's role in pleasure.

Help support your sisters, mothers and friends during their bleeding time. Talk to other women about the womb and its cycles with attention to the positive.

Chart your womb rhythms. Journal from your womb.

Notice your physical changes at ovulation.

How do these differ from the rest of your cycle?

Compare your womb chart rhythms with the phases of the moon.

Create a womb ritual or ceremony. An example:

A deep water womb ceremony for dreaming. May be used before bed.

Draw a warm bath. Add ¼ c. sea salt and a few drops of jasmine oil.

Light thirteen candles, one for each lunar month. (one candle will do but 13 is so pretty and symbolic)

Undress with intention. Remove all jewelry. Step in and soak.

As you relax, rest your right hand over your womb, your left hand over your heart. Breathe into your womb. Fill your womb and heart with light.

Imagine the glow spreading from your womb to your ovaries, from your heart to your breasts. Widen the glow through your body.

Exit the bath later with intention. As the water drains, allow your troubles and barriers to flow away.

Make a wish and blow out the candles. As you prepare to sleep, call on your angels and feel your womb as a wise source of love.

Begin a womb dream circle with other sisters or friends to share tools, insights and reconnect with traditional women's mysteries. It can be as simple as talking with your housemates or mother or daughters about your dreams, or asking about theirs.

Or you can gather with women at a regular time— moon cycle celebrations every month are ideal—and introduce readings, breathwork and self-care practices to each other in a teaching-learning community. All women have womb wisdom, all humans need it, and each of us has the potential to contribute, a story to share.

Uterine Self-Care Massage

Ancient Wisdom for Modern Practice

: Uterine Massage ~ also known as
: Maya abdominal massage :
is a timeless and gentle healing technique for accessing the creative and intuitive aspects of the sacred anatomy, as well as preventing and relieving reproductive health issues including:

- painful periods
- fibroids
- p.m.s.
  : and more :...

Massage brings increased circulation, energy and awareness to the pelvis. It is comforting and relaxing to give gentle attention to this seat of spiritual power.

To practice the technique is simple and accessible, however it is important to keep a few points in your awareness...

All Uterine Self-Care information courtesy of Deva Munay, LMT...

Uterine Self-Care Massage, ctd.
Cautions and considerations

(Because of cyclical changes in the) uterus-and each woman's unique condition- there are times when uterine self-care massage should be done <u>only</u> using extremely light or no pressure:

☆ Five days before your period
☆ During your period
☆ If you have an IUD
☆ If you have had surgery on or around the lower abdomen
☆ If you are pregnant
☆ If you are taking pain medications (that could cause you to not feel pain)

During these times, self-care may be a touch or hold of energy, sent through gentle hands to your womb. Listen to your body, she will tell you what she needs. ♡ ♡ ♡

Also: any type of self care massage, working deep in the body's core, can release deep emotions, memories and stories.

Please take the time to listen to your body, journal, breathe, take a walk and allow yourself to cry when needed. Drink plenty of water.

By experiencing fully the truths our bodies hold, by releasing the grief or anger we store inside, we are free to explore our bodies in joy and appreciation.

Never massage in a way that is painful, and consult your health care provider if you experience persistent pain - physically or emotionally - during massage. Supported healing is self-care too. Let your heart guide your process into greater love.

Self-Care Guidelines

Uterine Massage Std.

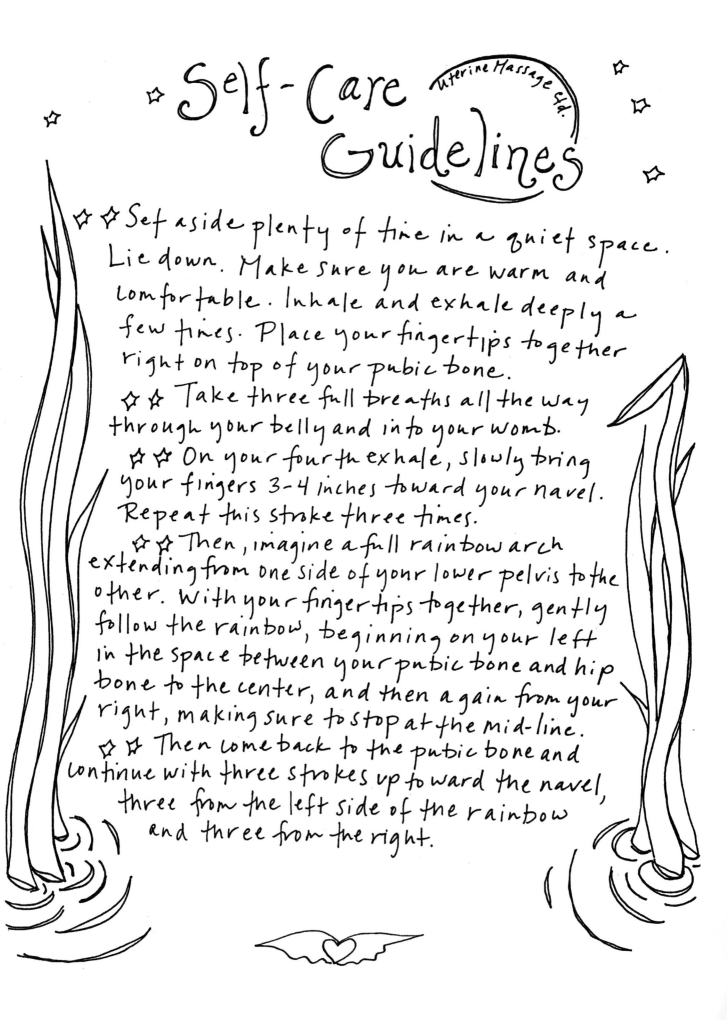

✩ ✩ Set aside plenty of time in a quiet space. Lie down. Make sure you are warm and comfortable. Inhale and exhale deeply a few times. Place your fingertips together right on top of your pubic bone.

✩ ✩ Take three full breaths all the way through your belly and into your womb.

✩ ✩ On your fourth exhale, slowly bring your fingers 3-4 inches toward your navel. Repeat this stroke three times.

✩ ✩ Then, imagine a full rainbow arch extending from one side of your lower pelvis to the other. With your fingertips together, gently follow the rainbow, beginning on your left in the space between your pubic bone and hip bone to the center, and then again from your right, making sure to stop at the mid-line.

✩ ✩ Then come back to the pubic bone and continue with three strokes up toward the navel, three from the left side of the rainbow and three from the right.

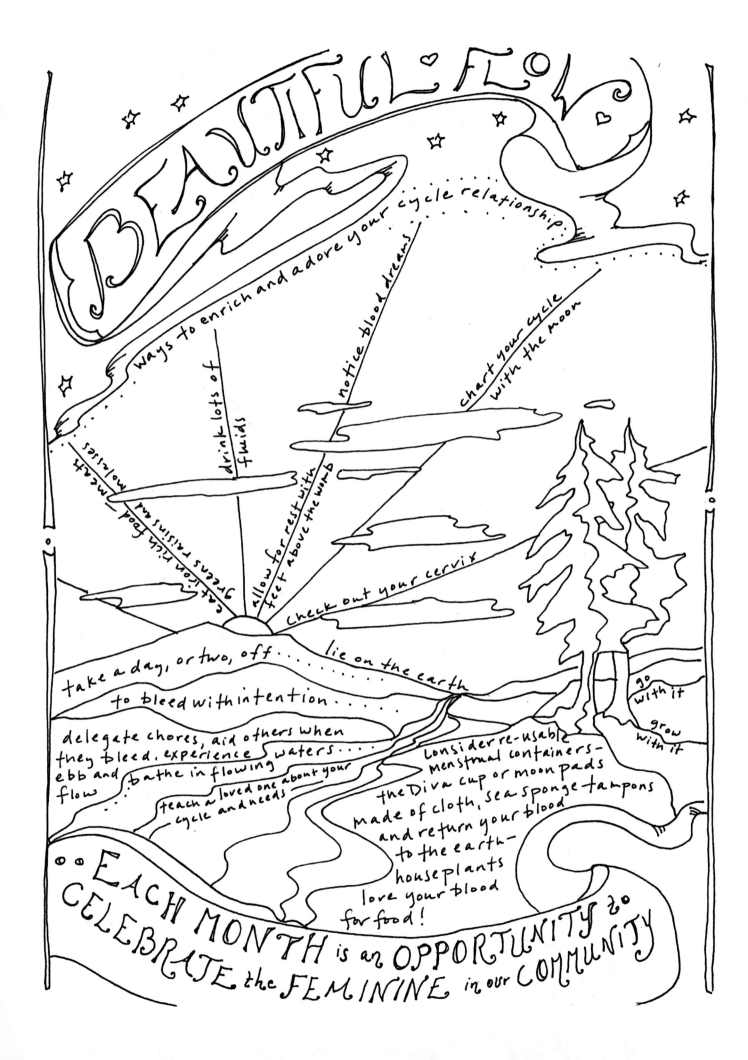

Blood · Root · Wisdom

A "what if" story

Once upon a time a girl was told, from the moment of her conception, that her body was precious and her blood sacred. At birth, the shared blood pulse through her umbilical cord is allowed to still before clamped and cut, her placenta blessed and used in ceremony. A circle of love surrounds her. She is taught strength but not fear, and her many teachers – men and women, mentors, relatives and friends – honor her growing autonomy with rituals to celebrate her. At the new moon she watches the women gather their life blood, blood of their womb, and return it with joy to the earth. She watches the bleeding women sing and rest, she learns their cycles and is not surprised, but eager and happy when one day she finds her blood has come. For days she learns the mysteries of transition, of womanhood. Her family and community gather to witness and bless her, as they will when she becomes a mother, as they will when she keeps her blood wisdom, an elder, a crone. For all of her bleeding days, in the whole of her living rhythm, she will honor her womb, she will lovingly collect her blood and return it to the earth. She will gather with other women. She will sing.

And she will tell her daughters and sons, from the moment of their conception, that their bodies are precious and their blood sacred. She will teach and celebrate her children. And they will tell their daughters and sons, from the moment of their conception, that their bodies are precious and their blood sacred.

Blood Love = Self Love

The more we can accept and love the unique powers of the feminine — both in physicality and principle — the more rich and joyful our lives become. To heal the feminine is to heal our culture, our planet, ourselves. Women's blood is <u>essentially</u> feminine, our cycles connect us powerfully with nature and each other. Yet, dominant culture reviles both.

BLOOD ACTION = CONSCIOUS

Bringing awareness to your "blood action" — how you treat your menstrual fluid — is an amazing and informative "gentle action" — culture and self transforming powerhouse without much personal effort.

Your blood is the blood of all women. It is the potential for all life in our species. It moves with rhythm, like moon and tide. Where does it go each month?

The whys of that revulsion are patriarchal, historical and many of the books listed in the Moon Divas works cited offer depth and root to this issue. Awareness is the key. How do <u>you</u> feel about menstrual blood? About your cycles and/or the cycles of others? Have you ever touched your own blood? What about the blood of another? How do you feel when you think about that? Why? What were you told when you began menstruating? Do you take birth control pills or hormones? What method of collection do you use? Why?

Consider answering some of these questions on the following page. Follow your intuition, draw a blood picture, tell a story about an experience with your blood that provoked a strong emotion — pain, happiness, desire, humiliation, ecstatic awareness.

· · · · · ·♡ ♥ ♡ ♡ ♥ ♡ ♥ · · · · · · ·

o The average woman will experience as many as 500 menstrual periods in her lifetime.
o She will cycle from menarche at around 12 to menopause at around 50.
o In her lifetime she will release 16 litres of fluid, roughly three times the amount of blood in her body.

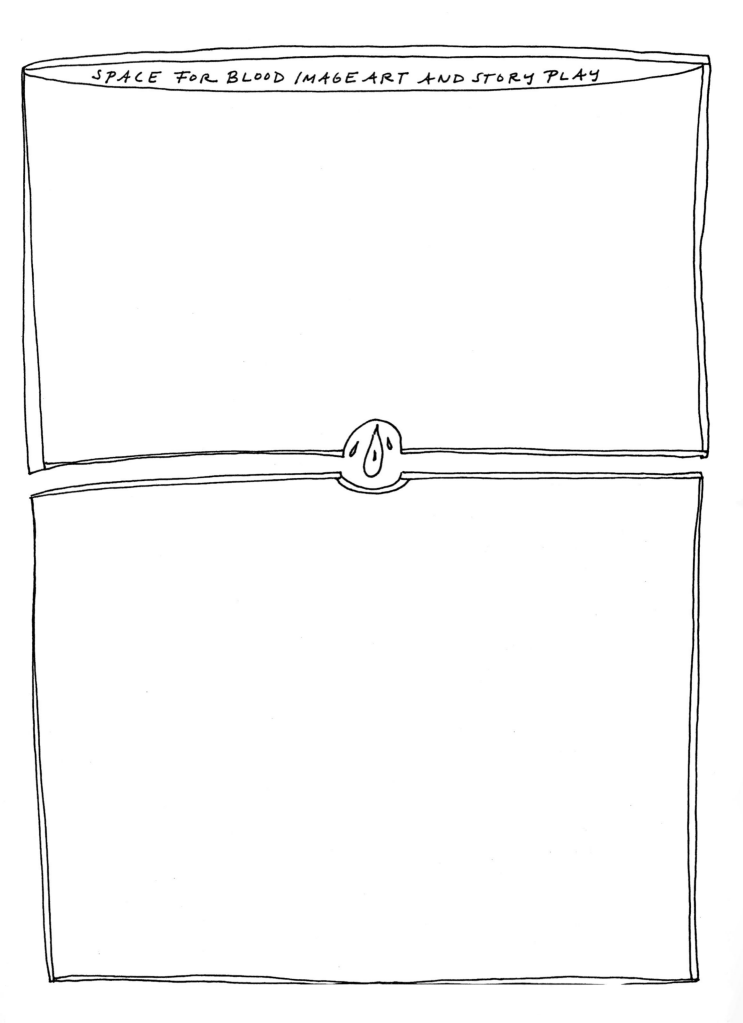

SPACE FOR BLOOD IMAGE ART AND STORY PLAY

SPACE FOR BLOOD IMAGE ART AND STORY PLAY

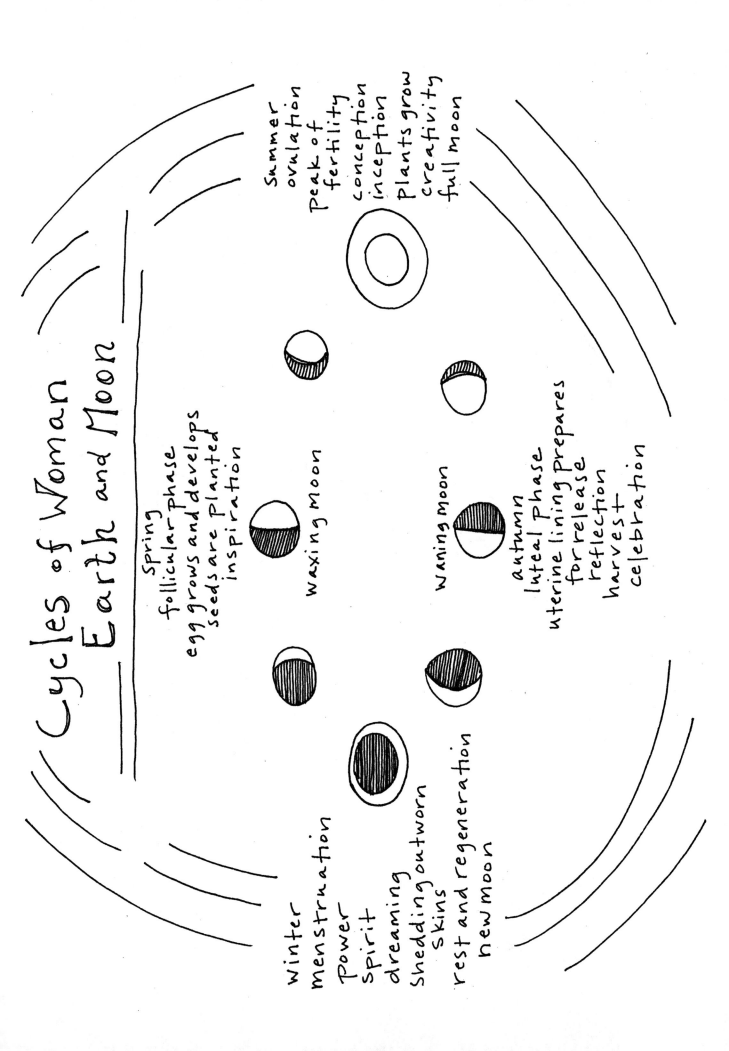

Cycles of Woman
Earth and Moon

Summer
ovulation
Peak of
fertility
conception
inception
Plants grow
creativity
full moon

Spring
follicular phase
egg grows and develops
seeds are planted
inspiration

waxing moon

waning moon

autumn
luteal phase
uterine lining prepares
for release
reflection
harvest
celebration

winter
menstruation
power
spirit
dreaming
shedding outworn
skins
rest and regeneration
new moon

A Cycle Chart for You!

If you are a menstruating woman, charting your cycle while getting to remember your womb has serious advantages.

First Day of Menstruation

Dates go here

You will begin to synchronize and understand what your body is telling you in each phase of your cycle. When we listen to our bodies and nourish our wombs, "symptoms" of many maladies may be alleviated.

The circular chart is numbered 1 through 30 around the edge.

For many women Days 10-19 are the most fertile. If you don't wish to conceive, take extra precaution before and during those days...

Every woman has a unique cycle, but most of us experience a 26-30 day cycle. The average is 28 days. After menstruation, at around day 10 in most cycles, the body begins to exhibit signs of fertility, and is preparing for ovulation at around day 14. This is your most fertile & creative time, a time of external shining energy, like the full moon. After ovulation, the energy moves inward, for a "period" of rest and reflection, the dark moon.

♡

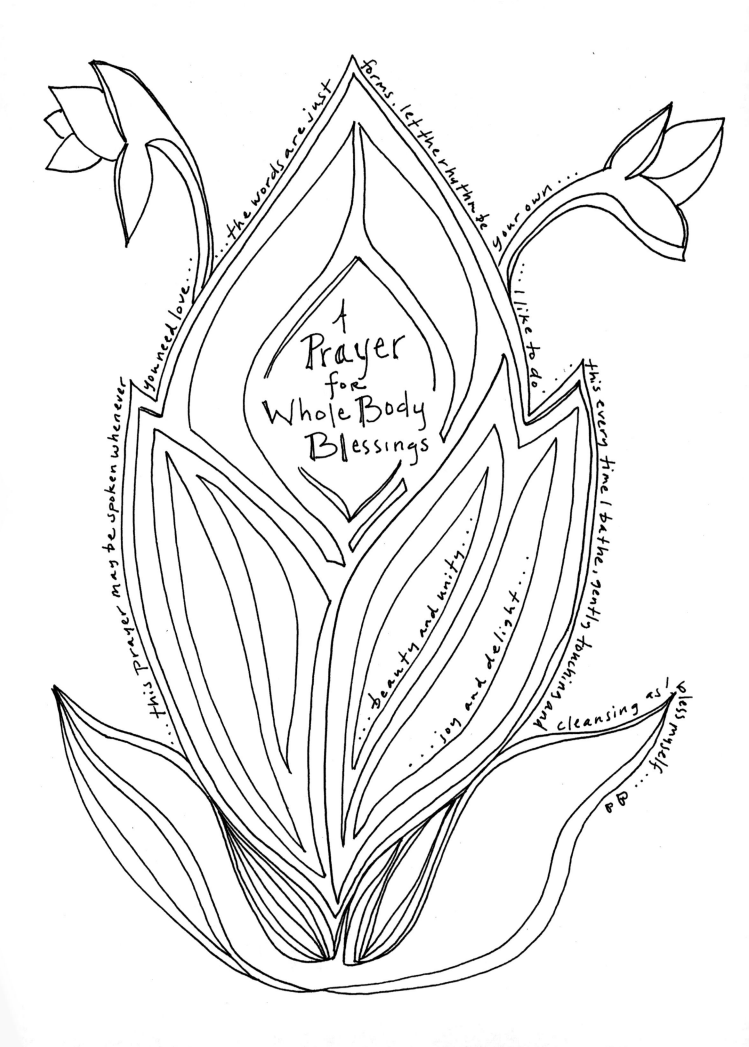

A Prayer for Whole Body Blessings

Mother Goddess who I
love, Creator, Universal One,
(insert your beloved life force name here),
I call on you in gratitude for this life and
all its beauties. I call on my ancestors, my
guardians and guides in the spirit of blessing, of joy
and remembrance for all that has come before. I offer
my heart in blessing and ask for your blessing in return.
Bless my eyes that I may see the wonder of the present.
Bless my lips that I may form words of love and reverence.
Bless my tongue that I may taste variety and be fully fed.
Bless my nose that I may recall the depth of the senses.
Bless my ears that I may appreciate the music of each day.
Bless my neck and shoulders, that they may carry my chosen weight.
Bless my arms that I may fully embrace the YES with love.
Bless my breasts that I may give and receive nourishment.
Bless my systems within, breath and pulse, miracles all.
Bless my belly that I may realize fulfillment.
Bless my side waists that make stretching into joy.
Bless my hips and pelvis, generous gravity, container of my holy womb.
Bless the womb and ovaries, gestation home, creative seeds.
Bless my ass that I may remember when to sit, when to jump.
Bless my vagina, her wisdom and her pleasure.
Bless my legs and feet, the journey is their strength.
Bless my hands, the channel for this art.
Bless my head, my brain, my mind and spirit.
Bless all that made way for this body
and this life, right now. May I go
forward in beauty, whole and
wholly loved.

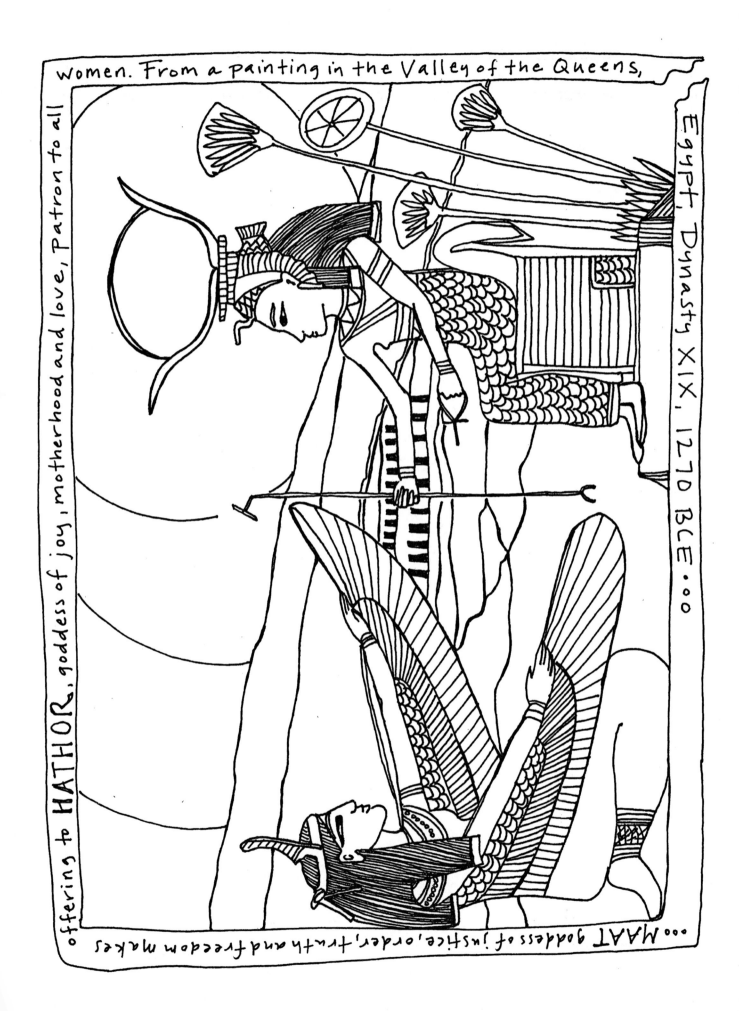

women. From a painting in the Valley of the Queens,

Egypt, Dynasty XIX, 1270 BCE...

offering to HATHOR, goddess of joy, motherhood and love, Patron to all

...MAAT goddess of justice, order, truth and freedom makes

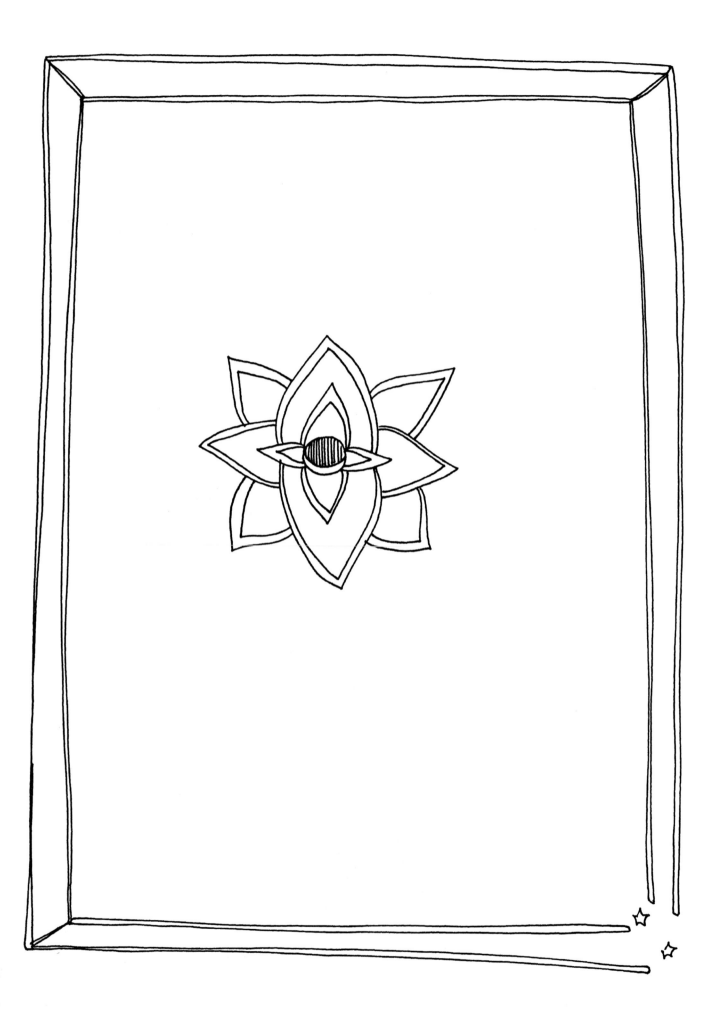

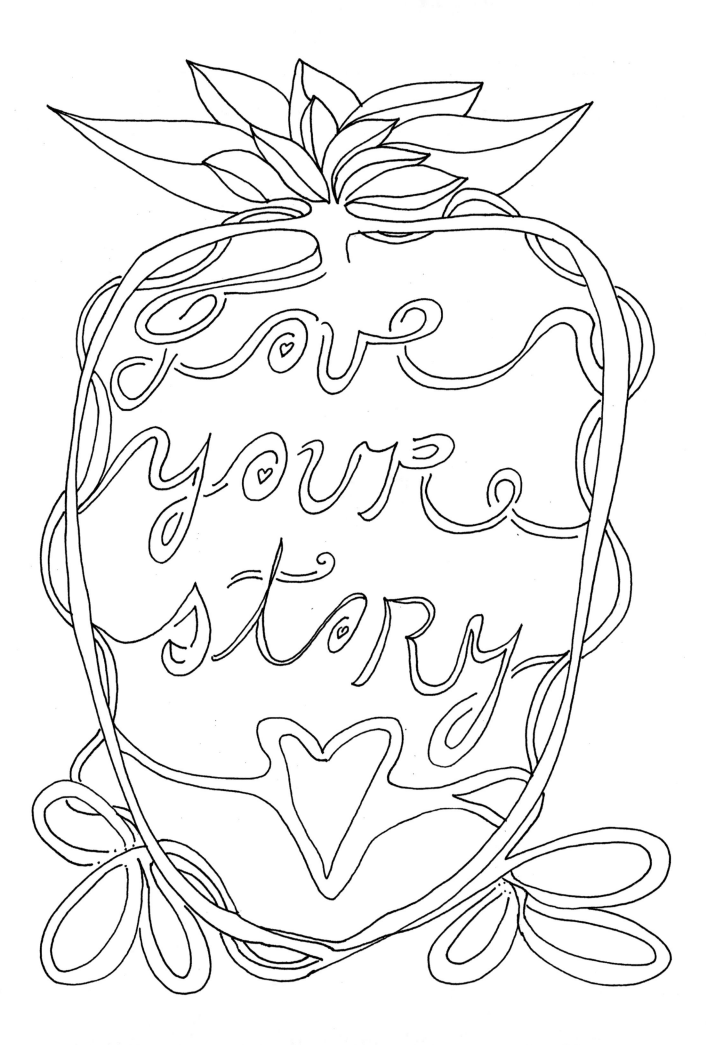

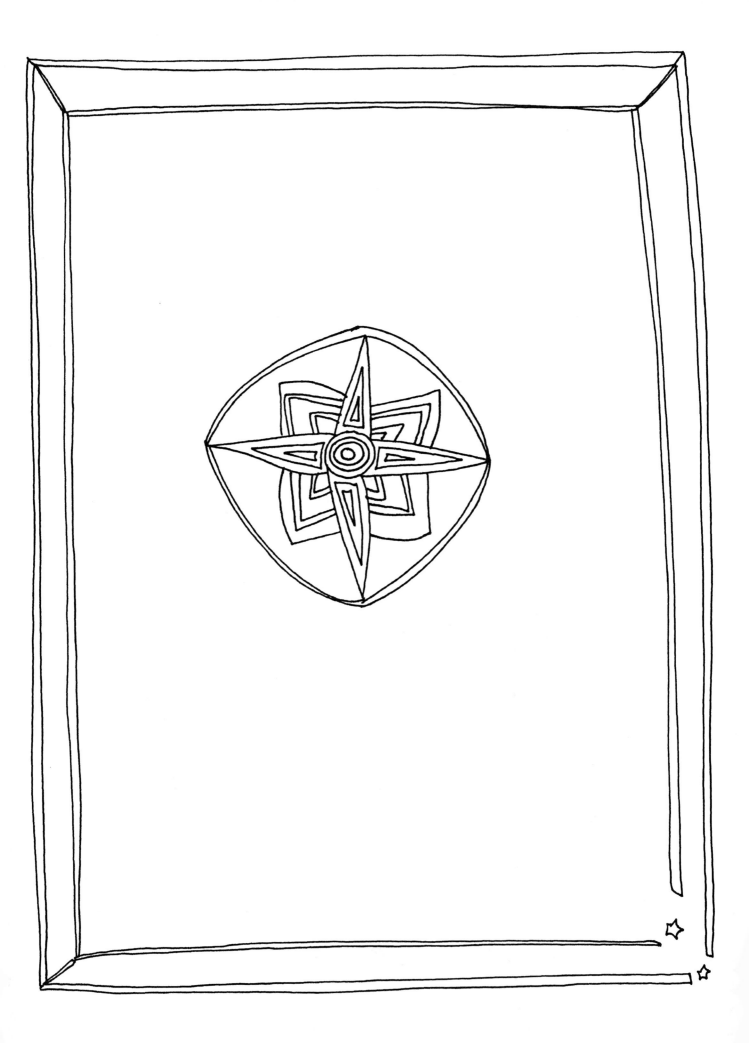

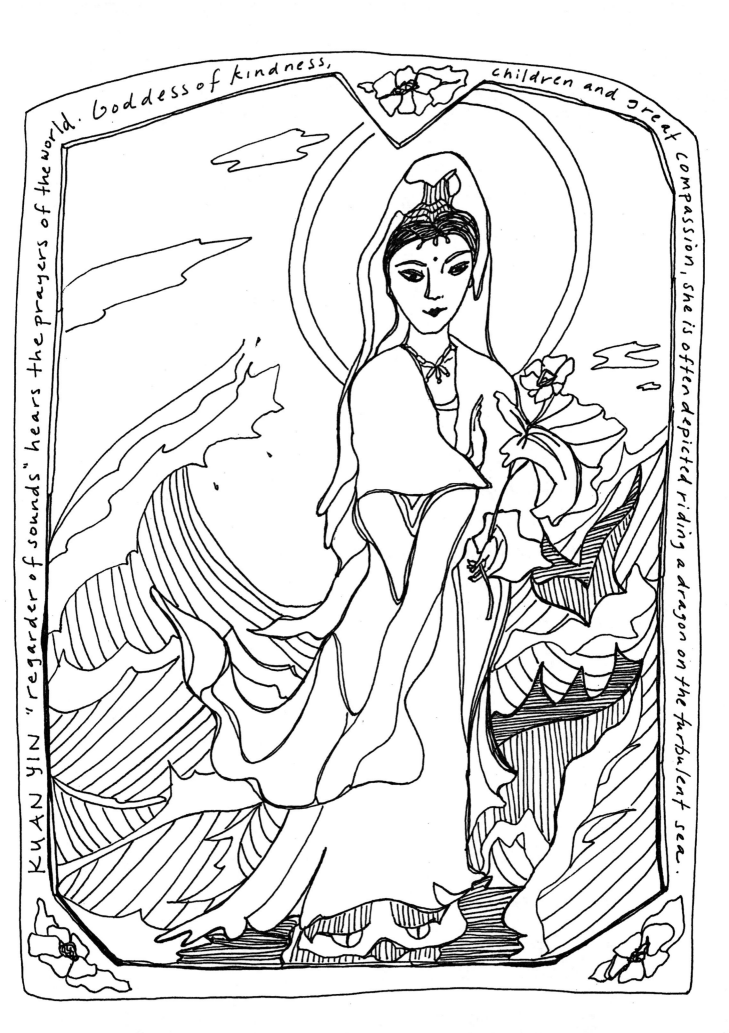

KUAN YIN "regarder of sounds" hears the prayers of the world. Goddess of kindness, children and great compassion, she is often depicted riding a dragon on the turbulent sea.

Stories
(to be read aloud)

Close your eyes and I will tell you a tale of the women who know their own stories. Stories of shelter, stories of strength, stories of faith and self-awareness. Stories of healing and hope and belonging. These stories are power, infused with the magic called creation. These stories make the world.

Sometimes these stories the women carried were not their own. Unconscious stories have power too, and may create the inner rhythm of many lives and days. These can be stories of lineage and culture... "you'll never be enough" is a common social story women carry. There are also stories of abuse, of victimization and trauma that can manifest with persistence through generations and block healing. There are stories thrust forward in the words and opinions of others, "you are so selfish, immature, silly, dumb... if you would only be different we could love and respect you." And then there are the stories of our secrets, which may, in hiding, fester a reality we believe we didn't choose.

But the women who know their own stories exercise a wonderful choice: They choose only those stories that belong to them wholly. They crack out into light their stories, lay them on the earth, follow their patterns to discover the stories' origin. They ask each story three questions:

☆ How are you serving me?
☆ What can I learn from you?
☆ Why should I keep you?

Letting go of old stories can be painful. There is often sadness, anger and fear in the void left by those stories. But the practice of story awareness, release and rebuilding is a beautiful challenge. Our hard stories teach and guide us. Discernment is knowing which stories we claim for their wisdom and which stories we've inherited or absorbed socially, but that hold no resonance at all.

Hard stories are meant to be shared, with sisters and daughters and friends. The power of storytelling is one of healing, integration and creative growth. Women create a vibrant world by sharing honest, conscious stories. ♡

Story Showing

.... may be practiced alone or with a group ...

☆ Story showing may be incorporated into any regular writing practice. Try it over a moon cycle, daily. How much energy moves as you witness your stories and claim what is yours?

☆ Story showing works with visuals too! Drawing, painting and collage are all ways to express and illuminate your story.

☆ Read your stories aloud, especially to people you love and trust (though reading to yourself is okay too). Watch the places where you self-censor or change the story in reading. Pay attention to the uncomfortable parts.

Light a candle and take a moment with your eyes closed to ground and center yourself. Breathe deeply. You may wish to acknowledge the four directions, the sky above you, the earth below. You may wish to call on spirit, angels, guardians and guides to witness and protect this journey. Ancestors are helpful here. Your body's chromosomes contain many stories. Many lives have come before you, and all of that living has brought you to this moment, this potential: You are a woman who will know her own story. And in this knowledge lies the hope for all women, past, present and future. Your story - the story you accept, honor, love, create and believe in - is the story of us all.

Now you are in sacred space. Gather your pen and paper. It is time to bring your inner narratives to light.

◊ Part 1 : The Old Story

☆ Think about the inner dialogue you hear when you are feeling down, vulnerable, insecure or just plain bad about yourself. Write it out for ten to twenty minutes. This might feel uncomfortable, or like a release. It may look silly or sad on the page (for example, "I'm so dumb I can't seem to do anything right"). That's okay.

☆ Part of the process is to keep writing. Don't censor, don't pause. Don't think, just write. Keep your pen moving. Write whatever comes to mind. If you start slowing down but know there is more, write a steady sentence (like "I don't know what else to write") until you reach the next level. What voices come through in the midst of the dialogue? Do you recognize anyone? Stop whenever you feel cleared, ready or done.

☆ When you are finished writing take a moment to breathe and stretch. Shake out your hands. Then read your work (I recommend reading aloud). Circle anything in the writing that feels like it has value, anything you wish to keep. Copy these words, phrases or sentences on a separate sheet of paper or next page.

☆ Take some space again and honor this story you have brought out to witness. How does your body respond to this story? How did it feel to write it? To read it? Use the next page to reflect on this portion of the process.

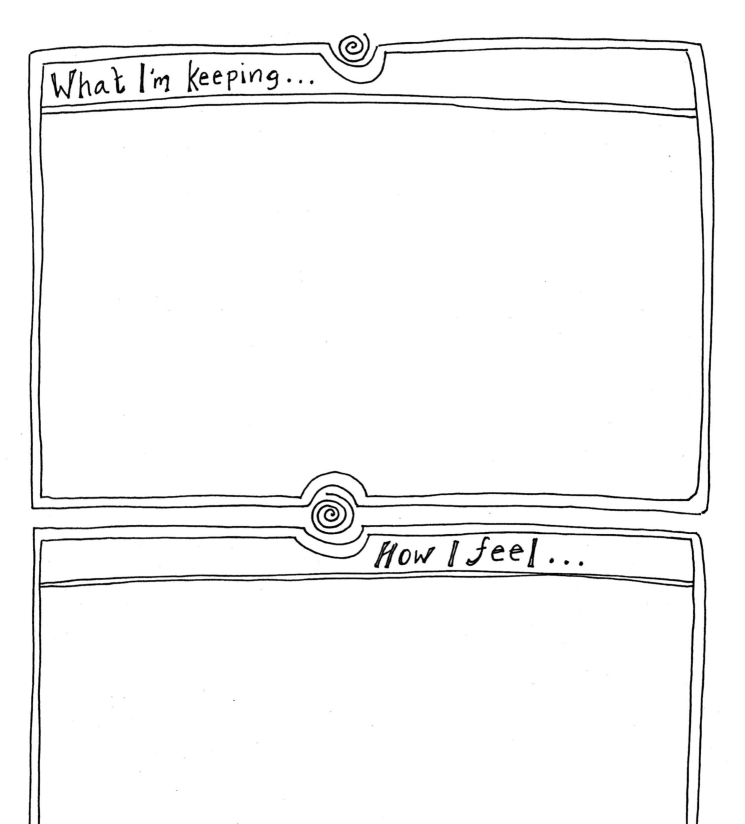

What I'm keeping...

How I feel...

Questioning the Old Story

You may wish to sit with the old story and the feelings it evokes for a while. But when you are ready it is time to question the story. As previously mentioned the following three questions are excellent to begin:
☆ How are you serving me? ☆ What can I learn from you?
☆ Why should I keep you? Additional questions might include the following: ☆ Where did you come from?
☆ How long have you been present? When did I first notice you? Who else do I know with a similar story? Write your answers to any of the above or your own unique questions in the space below.

Releasing the Old: Fire as Ally

Fire cleanses and purifies. What rises from the ashes literally in gardens, metaphorically or mythically in stories, is new growth. In the forest, fire clears deadwood and cracks seeds.

To release the old story you will need a place for safe burning (a fire pit, fireplace, barbecue, thick ceramic bowl or flower pot) and a source of flame.

note: respect and honor the power of fire. Never burn without full attention.

note: You may also complete this release by burying or composting your old story if fire is not an option.

☆ Examine the old story one last time. Then tear it into pieces. As you tear, speak aloud what you are letting go of. Fear? Secrecy? Shame? Be bold. Speak it.

☆ Then place the pieces in the burn receptacle. Set the old on fire.

☆ Watch it burn. Are there any words that catch your eye or linger? Bless them. Bless the old story. Let it go.

☆ When the ashes are cool place them on the earth or in a body of water. Then cleanse yourself with water, a bath or shower. The ocean, the rain. ♡

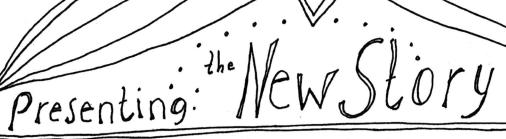

Presenting: the New Story

As the Phoenix is present, already, in the ashes, so is the New Story already inside you.

- She breathes every time you say, "If only...".
- She leaps each day you say, "I wish...".
- She begins with the answer to one holy question:

What kind of world do you wish to live in? ♡ _____

To begin the new story you must vision it deeply, as if it were already happening. Remember: your story carries incredible power. With the articulation of your vision you create the world for us all.

♡WRITING THE NEW STORY AS VISION♡

☆ Set aside a full hour for this exercise.
Begin by breathing and centering.
Quiet your mind.
Feel in to the joyful center of your heart.
Then start writing in first person present-tense:
"In the world I live in..."
Imagine this world deeply, use all of your senses to flesh out the details. Who are you in this world? What is the story that longs for you to live it? Keep your pen moving. Don't second-guess the strange, the wild, the power of the possible.

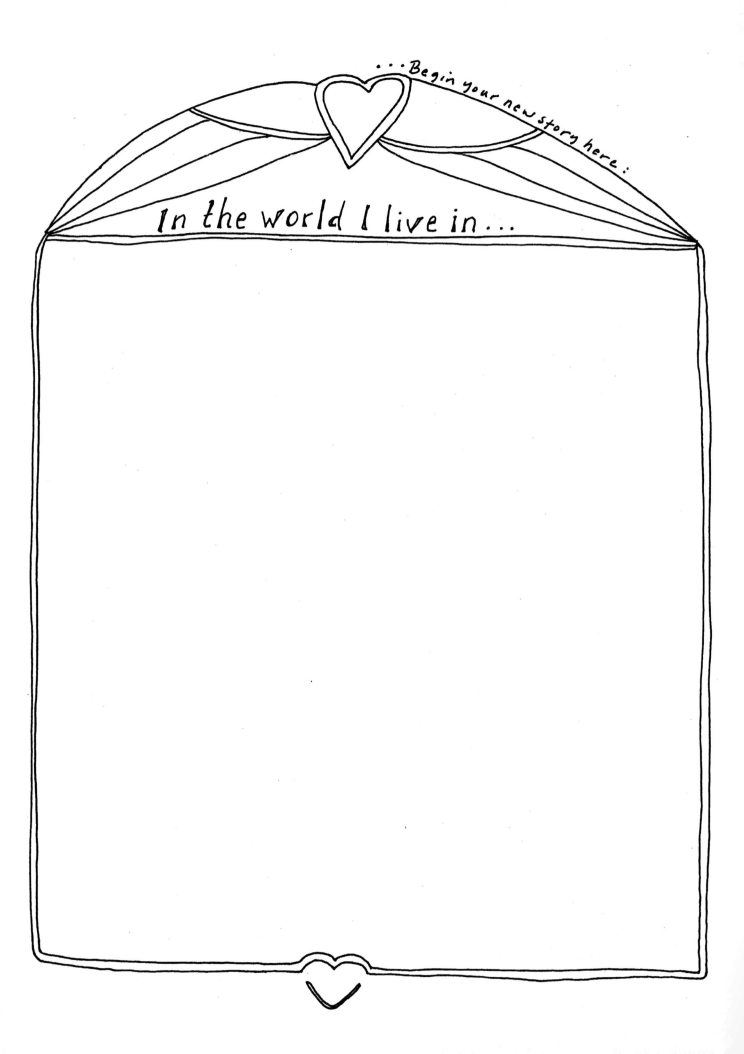

...Begin your new story here:

In the world I live in...

Other Entrances for the New Story

Exercise 1: Write a letter to yourself from the Divine — God, Goddess, Great Mystery, Universe, Higher Self — however you experience a higher compassionate essence.

Open your heart. Breathe. What does the greater creative power have to say to you? Does it address your present state, your past, your future purpose? How does this creator speak to you, through you?

Exercise 2: What nourishes you? Where do you feel your best — your strongest, most beautiful self?

Make a list of all the things that feed your body, your spirit, your heart.

What are the barriers to incorporating or experiencing this nourishment each day? List the barriers.

What supports do you have, internally or externally, for that which feeds you? List your supports.

Exercise 3: Write a story in first person present-tense ("I am") of your ideal day, a day where all your needs are met and you are fully supported. Go deep in your investigations, use all of your senses.

Notice the parallels between your support list and your story. How can you enhance or integrate these elements into your daily self-care practice? How can you bring more intention and awareness to the nourishment you already recieve?

Exercise 1: Letter from the Divine

Exercise 2: What Nourishes You?

NOURISHMENT	BARRIERS	SUPPORT

Exercise 3: An Ideal Day

Parallels with support list:

Ideas on how to integrate more:

The new story requires love and attention. It must be <u>practiced</u>, not just recited. It is a dynamic living being, your creation. What nourishes you, feeds the new story. Regular self-care and affirmation, ritual and prayer, strengthen the new into being.

Sometimes we will resist the new story. By recognizing and surrendering those elements we are attempting to manipulate (our fears, our image of how it "should" be) we continue to supply the new story with room to grow.

What three things can you surrender? Leave them in the jar!

1.

2.

3.

Create a Prayer Box or Wish Jar......

What remains? What are you grateful for? Write it here:

The New Story Requires Self-Love ♡ ♡ ♡

♡ Ten things I Love About ♡
♡ ♡ Myself ♡ ♡
Right Now :

1.

2.

3.

4.

5.

6.

7.

8.

9.

10.

☆11.

☆12.

☆13.

keep going !! you are amazing !!!

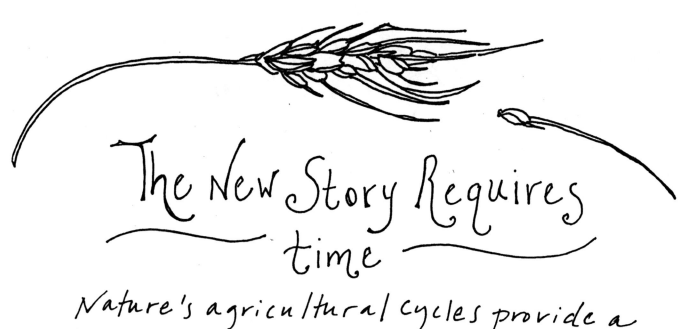

The New Story Requires time

Nature's agricultural cycles provide a metaphorical structure for understanding, for living, our lives. We reap what we sow. The new story is a seed planted within, perhaps long ago... a two thousand year old date palm sprouted from its seed when given soil, water, food and light. Patient tending is required of all growing things. Love, deep nourishment and time heal, restore and foster the cycles of living.

Love the seed. Love yourself for the planting. Love the moment of beginning, now, the journey of your growth.

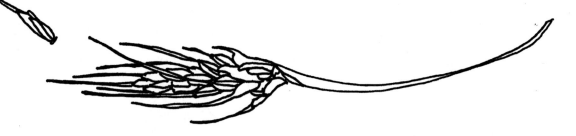

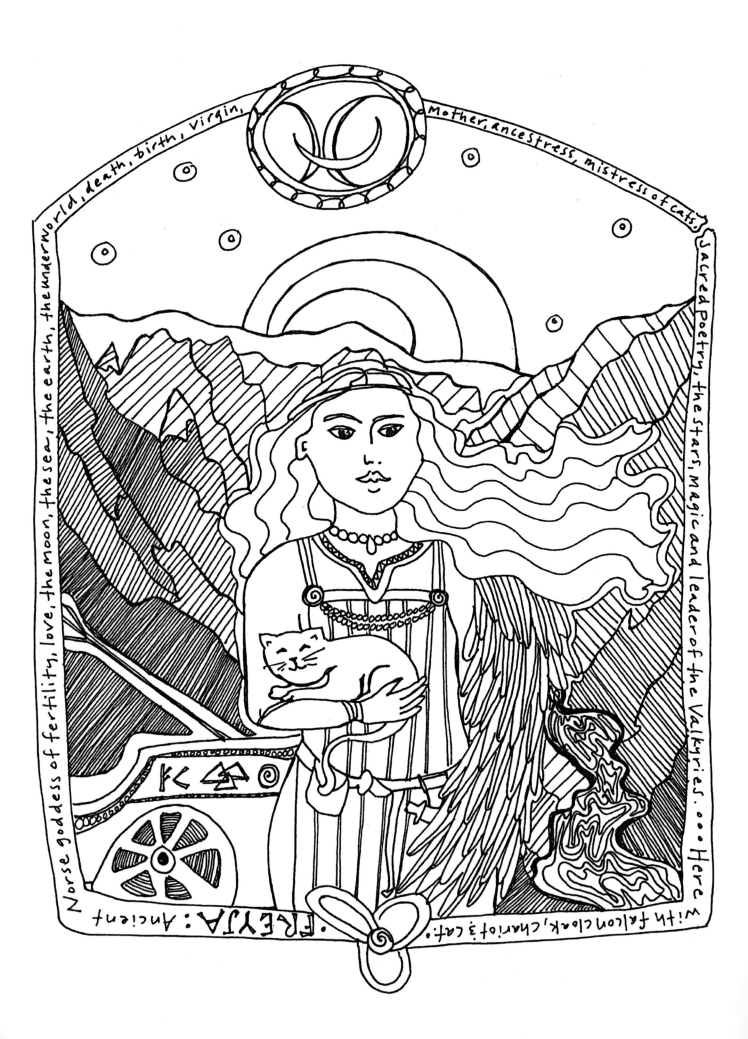

Norse goddess of fertility, love, the moon, the sea, the earth, the underworld, death, birth, virgin, mother, ancestress, mistress of cats, Sacred poetry, the stars, magic and leader of the Valkyries....Here with falcon cloak, chariot & cat.

FREYJA: Ancient

SACRED Story

Myth, Legend, Saga, Fable, Fairy Tale, Allegory, Metaphor, Shapeholder

Once Upon a Time

we Moon Divas decided to play dress up. After releasing the old story and writing the new, Deva and I both realized there were some tools we needed to develop, some qualities we needed to enhance in order to fully embody the new story. We decided to choose a goddess persona to enact as we went out for dinner, just for fun. I chose the Norse Goddess Freyja for her boldness, her beauty and her stories which told of a powerful feminine presence. Deva chose the Hindu Goddess Durga, a peaceful warrior gifted with twelve magical implements, one for each of her twelve hands.

We looked up the goddess' images and myths, their symbols and correspondences. We dressed the part, adorned ourselves and

headed out to meet what would be an
unforgettable night. We were both making
choices from a much bigger place, asking
ourselves if a Goddess would be content with
the wrong order, or if a Goddess would worry
if someone didn't return a phone call. I felt
stretched and full, calm and delighted. I
realized this Goddess, this greater aspect,
the Divine feminine, has always been
in me. She is me. Spiritually, mythically,
archetypically, we all may access this greater,
this pantheon of stories, personas, essences
that have described women's experience
and potential for thousands of years.
We are not alone. Our ancestral heritage
waits for us to be curious, to call Her name.
   Since that night Deva and I have
worked with many women, bringing this
experiment into a larger venue is enlivening,
empowering and beautiful to witness. We have
sat for Goddess tea and Goddess lunches
where each woman present dresses

Sheelah-na-gig REA Minerva ISIS Hutk/x Chel Athena
Vesta Erzulie RHEA Minerva ISIS Hutk/x Chel Athena
Aphrodite Isamba Spider Woman SOFHIA Chup Mut Holda
ATHENA Inanna SARASVATI Aditi Ostara Hecate BRIGIT Astraea Tamra Pele
Olwen Irene BERCHTA Cybele Ostara Hecate
Changing Woman Mene
Mache Amatis Nat
Juno SAULE
Dag

the part of one of our
ancient mothers. We research and
tell the stories, we invoke through seasonal
ritual the process of becoming, of revealing
the Goddess within. In the welcoming of
the feminine in her many guises, there is
room for all we are, and all we wish to be.

For thousands of years the Goddess
was celebrated, central to and along with
God in many — perhaps most — diverse cultures.
She is still central to the spirit of millions
today, her names and shapes familiar on
every continent. Her absence creates more
absence in every woman who looks for a
model, a story, of range and power.

When we reclaim the vast stories of
the feminine divine, when we see her — even
metaphorically — as ourselves, when we
share knowledge and beauty with other
women, we do grow. She becomes more than
a persona — a mask — and instead is an
intricate, inextricable part of
what we always have been.

Kishi-Mujin Pajan Yan Quan Yin
Tara HALTIA
Lilith Thestan Oshun
Kali Ma Idun Edna Persephone HYBELA Oya ZHINU HATHOR Baba Yaga DANU
Bast Mary CIMIDYE Demeter Bean Woman Ix Chebel Yax Fortuna
maia Saki Yama-Hime

✫ Inviting the Goddess to Play ✫

Do you choose a Goddess or does the Goddess choose you? Both. Or, at least, try both. There are many beautiful Goddess Oracle Cards, and books, like 365 Goddess by Patricia Telesco or The Book of Goddesses by Kris Waldherr, allow the perusal of a number of symbols and stories. You can choose consciously, based on the qualities you wish to embody, or unconsciously with the divinitory art of stichomancy (put your finger blindly in a closed book), or by drawing a card. I like to ask: What Goddess do I need to work with?

Once you've chosen, the fun begins. You may wish to conduct some inquiry as to the Goddess's history. You might like to conduct a ritual — a bath or other cleansing — to invite the Goddess in. Have fun with the initiation. See what develops.

Involving other women in this experience is incredible. Deva and I still call each other Freyja and Durga, three years later. I've come to recognize Freyja as a relative. Her presence is palpable and she is always calling me to be courageous.

Through this book I have included images of some of my favorite Goddesses. On the following pages I hope you will record your goddess experiments, complete with illustration. You may also wish to draw on feminine figures from your own spiritual tradition. My Great Grandmother, Nana Louise, was the first person I knew who revered a female image. The statue was in the center of her living room surrounded by candles and flowers. She was the Virgin Mary and my Nana said she prayed to her for strength.

Your First Goddess

·A PHOTO· ·A DRAWING· ·A SYMBOL· ·A SHRINE·

Healing with Myth and Story

We may all be, at various times, alone — or at least feel alone — in our journey. Transition & passage, sometimes requires time or space alone, and this can be the healthy sort of quiet or room needed for transformation. But isolation is another matter. Sometimes when we are traveling through difficult, uncharted territory, we can seem uniquely, totally, sealed off from our friends and family and the social stories that have sustained us.

When I divorced and moved away from my young children to find work, I quickly became unlike any woman I had ever known. My children — particularly my daughter — and I struggled with trying to find forms, answers, advice for what could work in our situation. There were few. My pain, guilt and unknowing felt endless.

As with so much of this Moon Divas work, the answers I sought came, both from without and within. I prayed for guidance, and my daughter came home with the story of Demeter and Persephone from the library. We read it together, then looked at each other. "Mama, that's like you and me!" my daughter said.

In this version of the powerful and timeless story of maternal separation, Persephone is happy and powerful as the queen of the underworld. And Demeter uses the time in Persephone's absence to catch up on some much-needed rest. They use their time apart to deepen and enrich their lives.

Knowing that thousands of forms exist, echoing our literal and metaphorical stories, is empowering. We are not alone in our trials. And once we seek a form or myth to work with, sometimes the honest opening of our story into a greater light can embolden us to share with others. In telling my story I have found others, mothers and children both, living full lives richly apart. We share, we open, we heal.

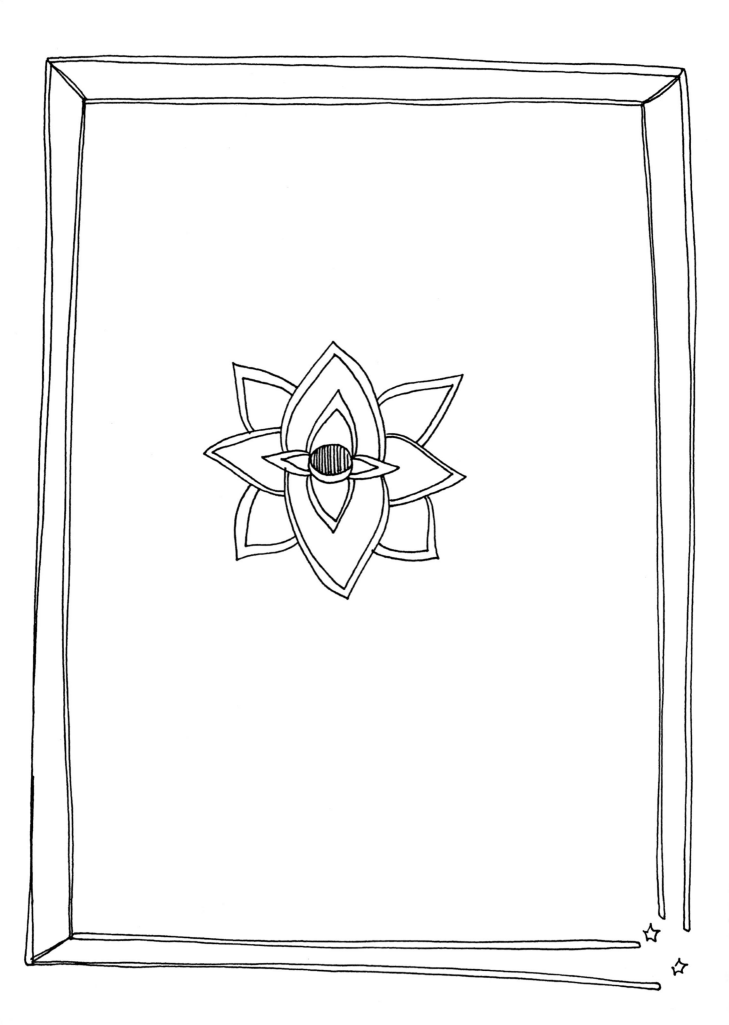

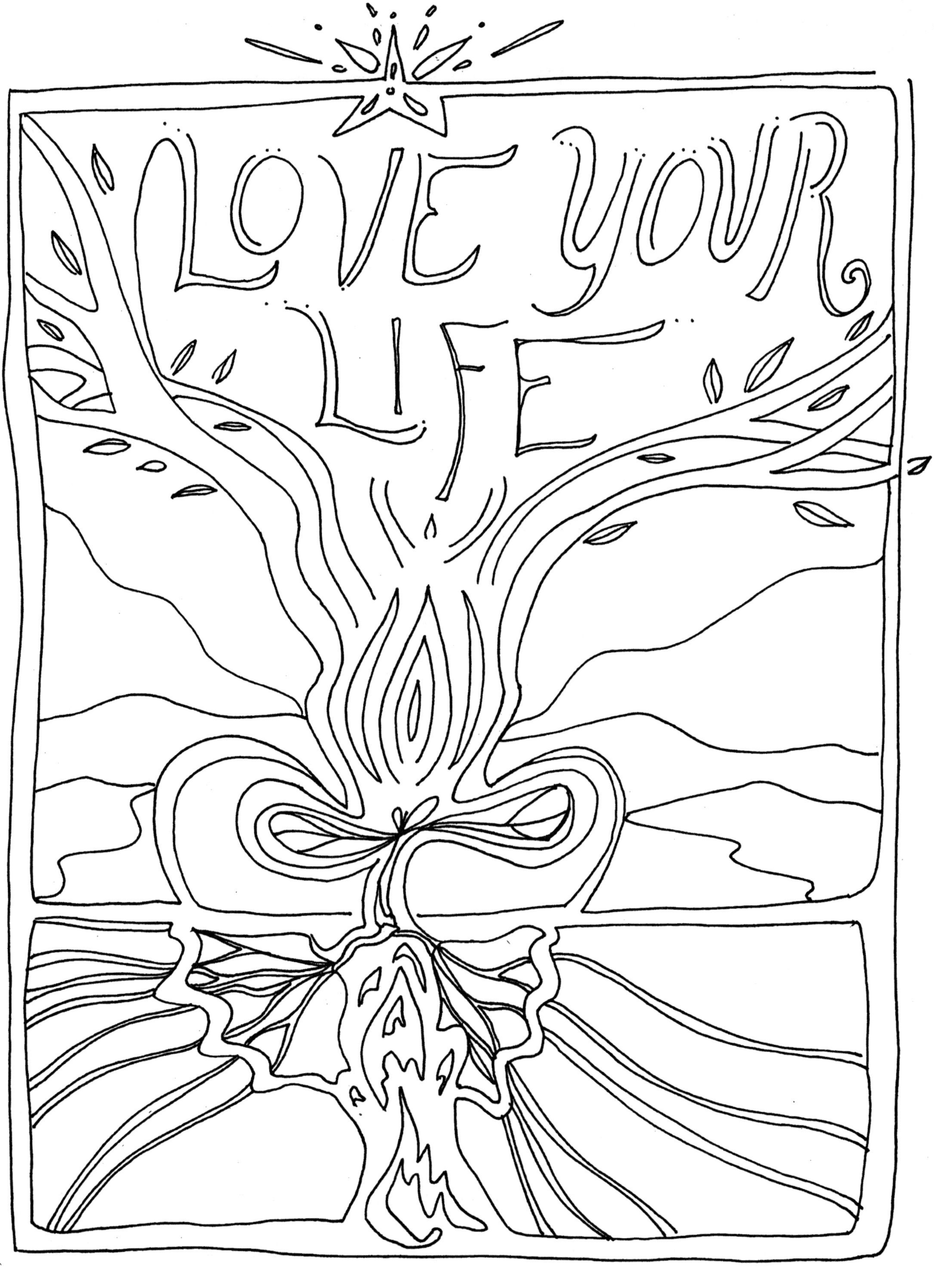
LOVE YOUR
LIFE

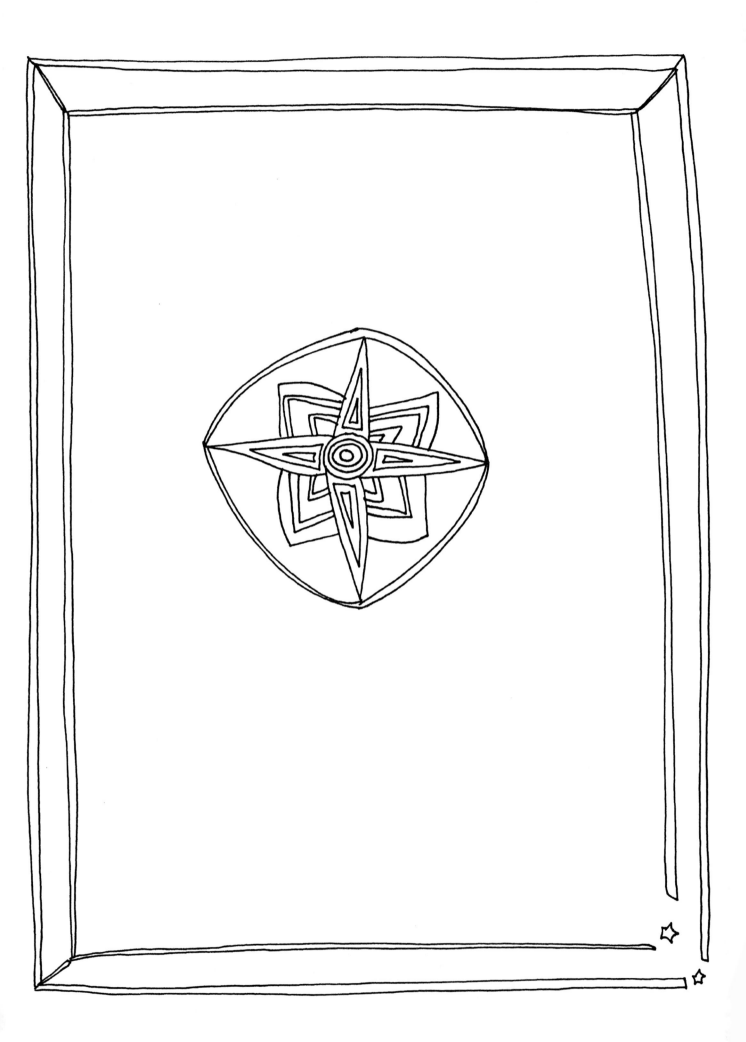

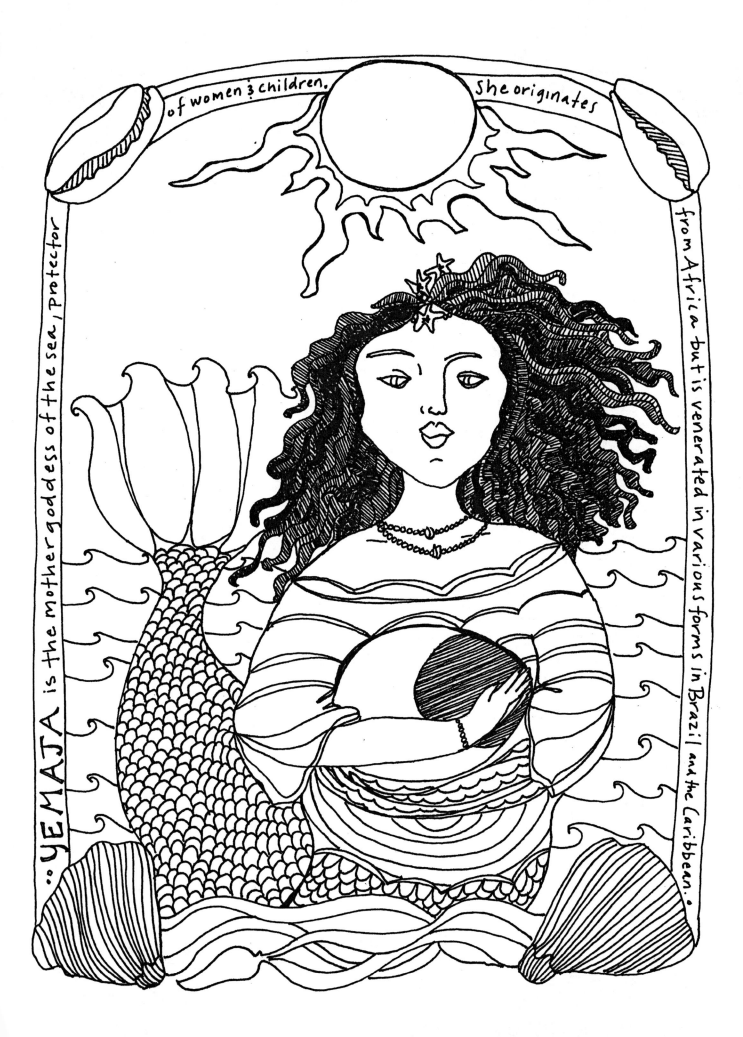

...YEMAJA is the mother goddess of the sea, protector of women & children. She originates from Africa but is venerated in various forms in Brazil and the Caribbean.

Sister Circles
CRAFTING COMMUNITY & HOLDING SPACE

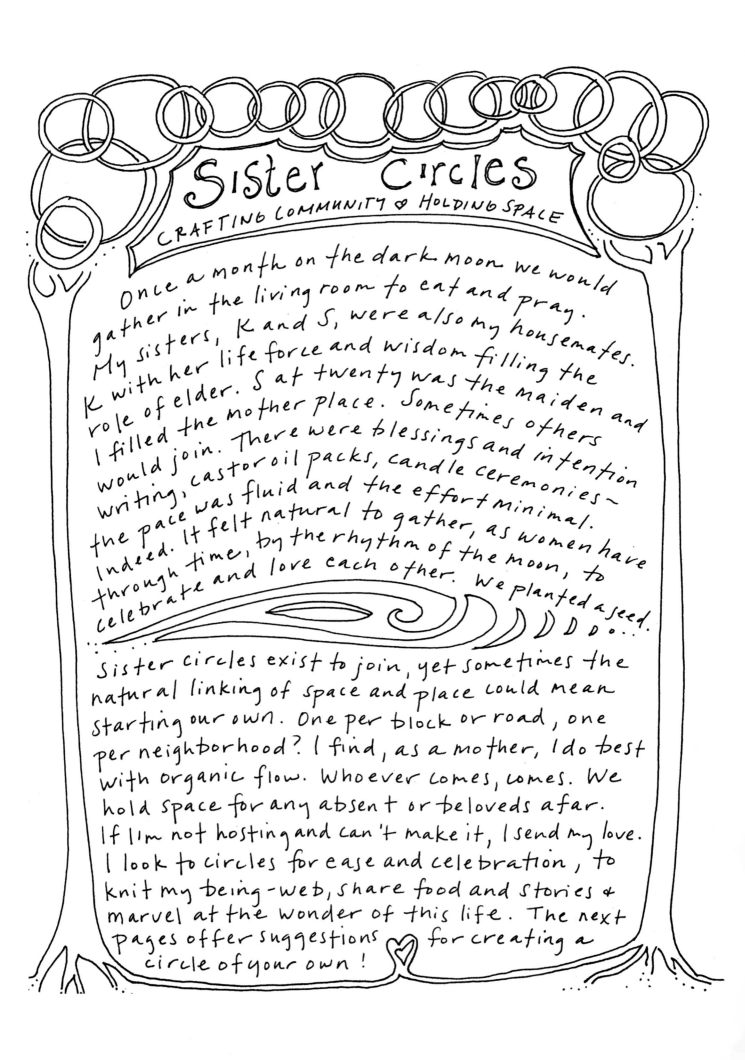

Once a month on the dark moon we would gather in the living room to eat and pray. My sisters, K and S, were also my housemates. K with her life force and wisdom filling the role of elder. S at twenty was the maiden and I filled the mother place. Sometimes others would join. There were blessings and intention writing, castor oil packs, candle ceremonies ~ the pace was fluid and the effort minimal. Indeed. It felt natural to gather, as women have through time, by the rhythm of the moon, to celebrate and love each other. We planted a seed.))) o...

Sister circles exist to join, yet sometimes the natural linking of space and place could mean starting our own. One per block or road, one per neighborhood? I find, as a mother, I do best with organic flow. Whoever comes, comes. We hold space for any absent or beloveds afar. If I'm not hosting and can't make it, I send my love. I look to circles for ease and celebration, to knit my being-web, share food and stories & marvel at the wonder of this life. The next pages offer suggestions ♡ for creating a circle of your own!

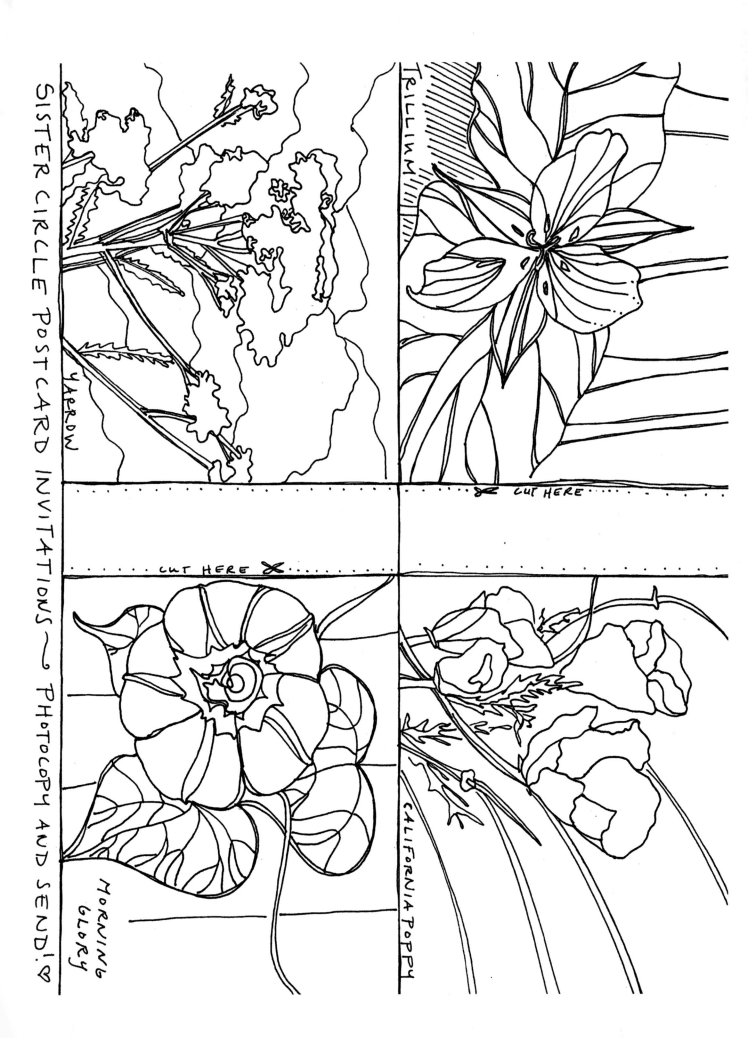

SISTER CIRCLE POSTCARD INVITATIONS— PHOTOCOPY AND SEND! ♥

YARROW

TRILLIUM

✂ CUT HERE

CUT HERE ✗

MORNING GLORY

CALIFORNIA POPPY

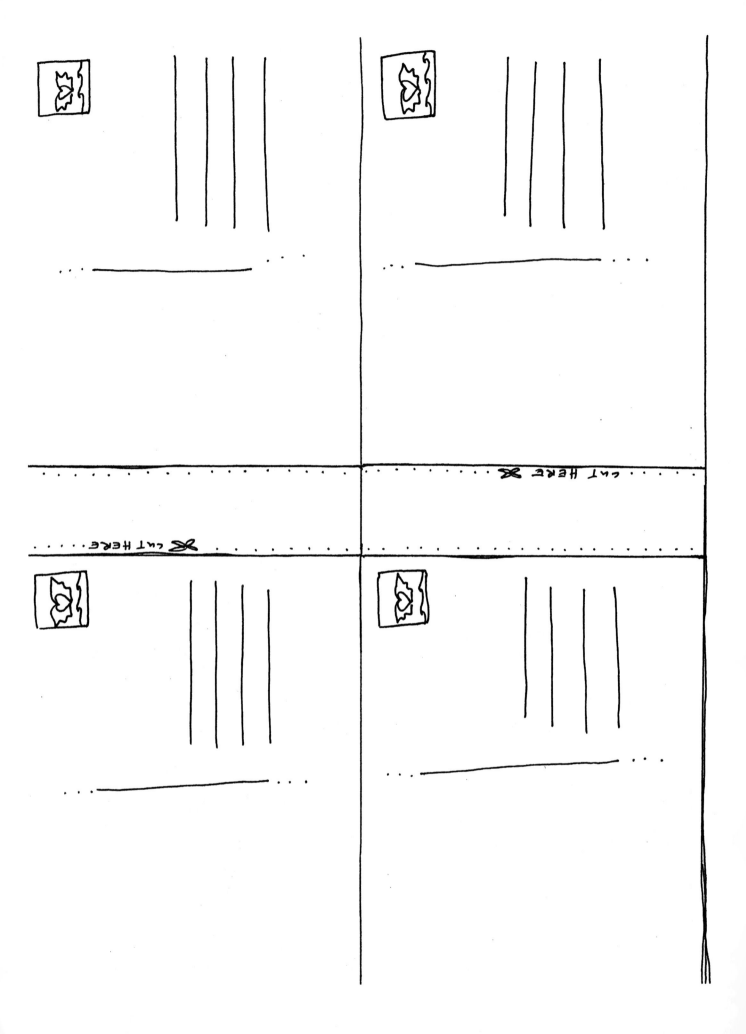

cut HERE ✂

✂ cut HERE

PLANNING IS...

✩ Best in partnership. Do you have a friend, neighbor, relative or co-worker willing to support the initial event? Make it fun!

✩ Important, but try to make room for spirit, too. Micro managing wears us out and usually doesn't serve the whole. Keeping the first meetings simple allows for the group to become what it needs to be.

CONSIDER COORDINATING

✩ specifics: time, place, duration and food (pot-luck is always wonderful). 2-3 hours may be plenty to start.

✩ an ice breaker (examples below) to sluff off rowdy nerves.

✩ a gift or token for all to go away with. Simple and inexpensive items can also be powerfully symbolic: seeds (see intentions exercise) shells, stones, etc.

....° SISTER CIRCLE ....
STARTUP SWEETS

TRUST THAT...

✩ Whoever is supposed to be present will arrive. A "circle" can be carried with any number as long as it is done with intention.

✩ The circle is more than the sum of its parts. Elaborate ritual or pagentry are not essential to cultivate nurturing and growth in those present. Sometimes knowing when to do nothing at all can make room for what is necessary.

MAYBE TRY...

✩ Having participants stand in a circle and close their eyes, breathing together before starting on introductions.

✩ Ask everyone to tell a story about their name, or

✩ name their feminine lineage as far back as they can remember, or

✩ tell a story about a time they felt good being female, or

✩ list ten things they love about themself...

A talking stick can be a useful tool for reminding the circle to be respectful of the speaker. Consider a sharing circle at the end too!

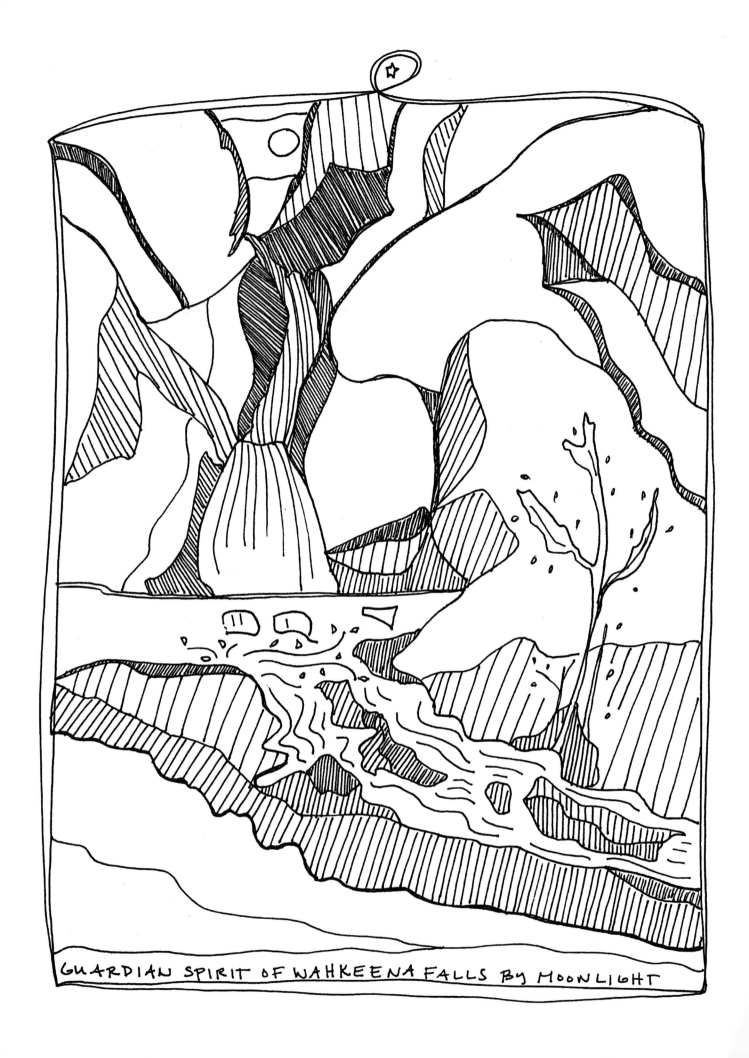

GUARDIAN SPIRIT OF WAHKEENA FALLS BY MOONLIGHT

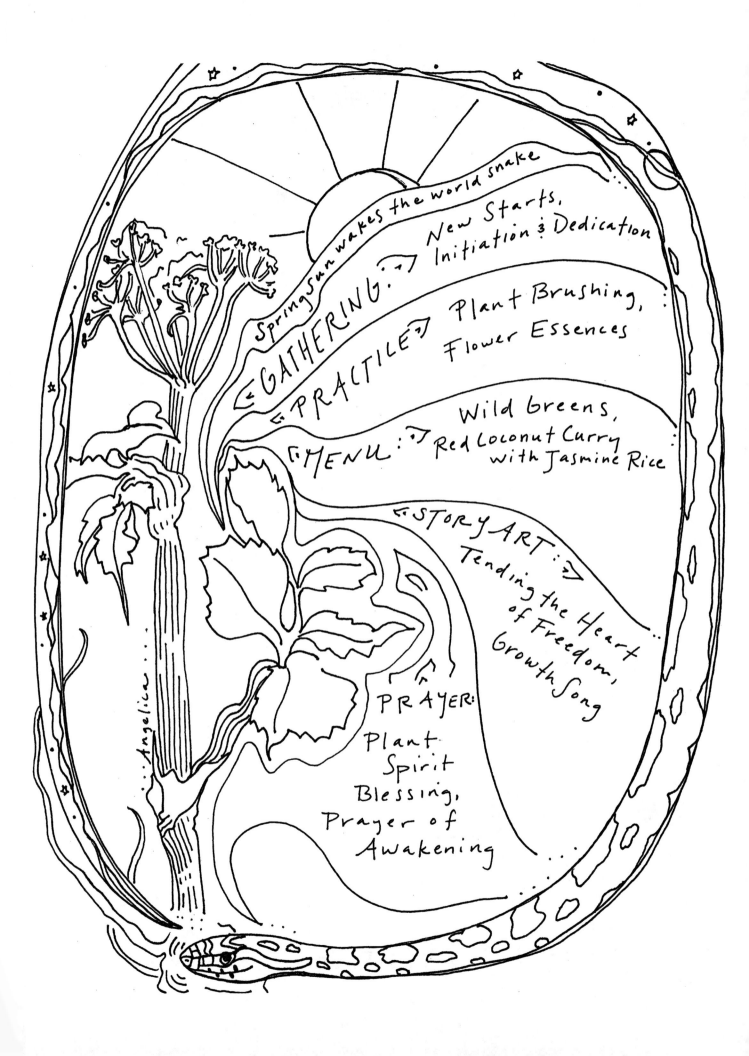

Spring sun wakes the world snake

GATHERING → New Starts, Initiation & Dedication

PRACTICE → Plant Brushing, Flower Essences

MENU → Wild Greens, Red Coconut Curry with Jasmine Rice

STORY ART → Tending the Heart of Freedom, Growth Song

PRAYER: Plant Spirit Blessing, Prayer of Awakening

...Angelica...

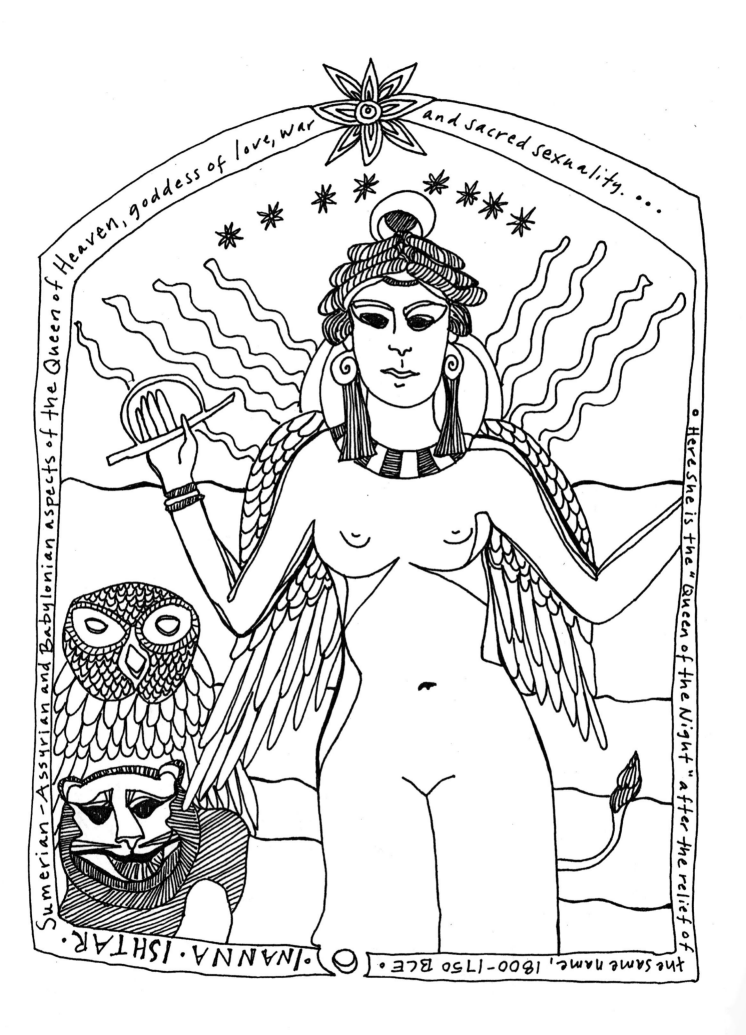

Sumerian—Assyrian and Babylonian aspects of the Queen of Heaven, goddess of love, war and sacred sexuality. . . . • Here she is the "Queen of the Night" after the relief of the same name, 1800–1750 BCE • •INANNA·ISHTAR•

WAKENING AND ABUNDANCE

TENDING THE HEART OF SPRING

"WAKE UP, WAKE UP!" my favorite birds return to Northern Oregon in February, right around the cross-quarter day between the winter solstice and the Equinox. Days inch longer, catkins hang on hazel and alder, seeds split and root, the fields glow low rainy green and stretch skyward. All this before the blooming. This initiative and determined energy, this is spring, too, in your body and psyche. It is through dedication and commitment to the process of our growth that we nurture the eventual split of bud, the full flowering.

Spring Circle Suggestions:

✿ Ceremony of initiation for those entering a new phase of life

✿ dedication circle to encourage new directions or growth

✿ seed and plant exchange garden planning symbolism intentions planting

✿ singing circle in beautiful dresses invoking the sun (think "O Heavenly Day," "Uncloudy Day," "Here Comes the Sun")

✿ spring-themed pot luck and wild plant tasting: dandelions, chickweed, violets...

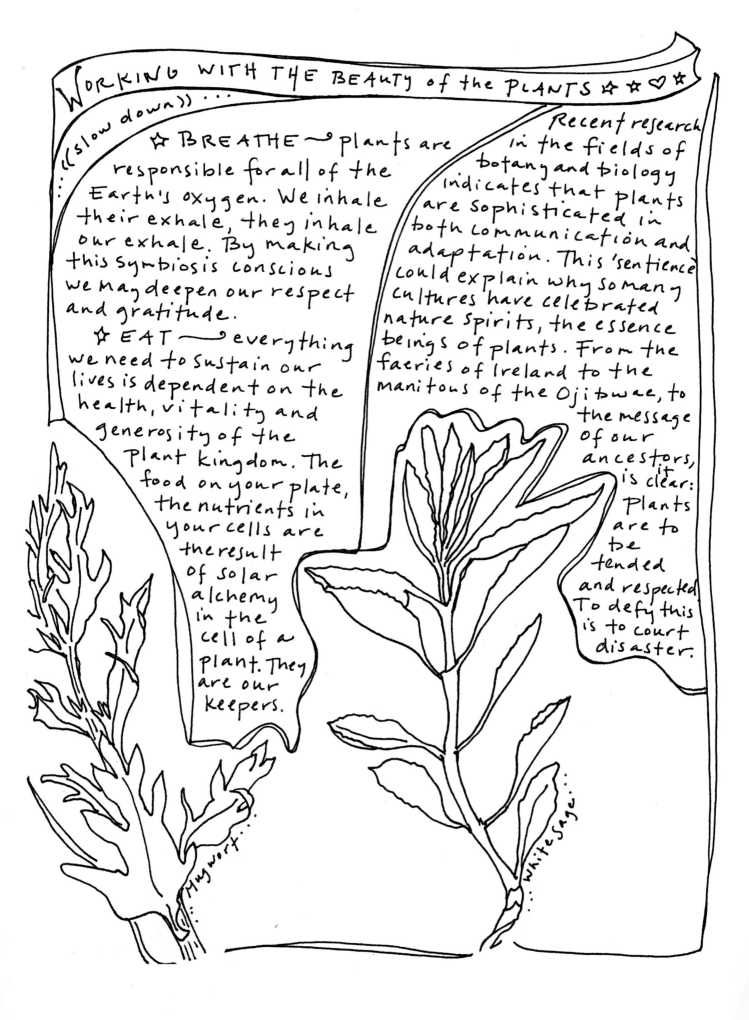

((slow down)) ...

✿ BREATHE ~ plants are responsible for all of the Earth's oxygen. We inhale their exhale, they inhale our exhale. By making this symbiosis conscious we may deepen our respect and gratitude.

✿ EAT ~ everything we need to sustain our lives is dependent on the health, vitality and generosity of the Plant kingdom. The food on your plate, the nutrients in your cells are the result of solar alchemy in the cell of a plant. They are our Keepers.

Recent research in the fields of botany and biology indicates that plants are sophisticated in both communication and adaptation. This 'sentience' could explain why so many cultures have celebrated nature spirits, the essence beings of plants. From the faeries of Ireland to the manitous of the Ojibwae, to the message of our ancestors, it is clear: Plants are to be tended and respected. To defy this is to court disaster.

Mugwort

white sage

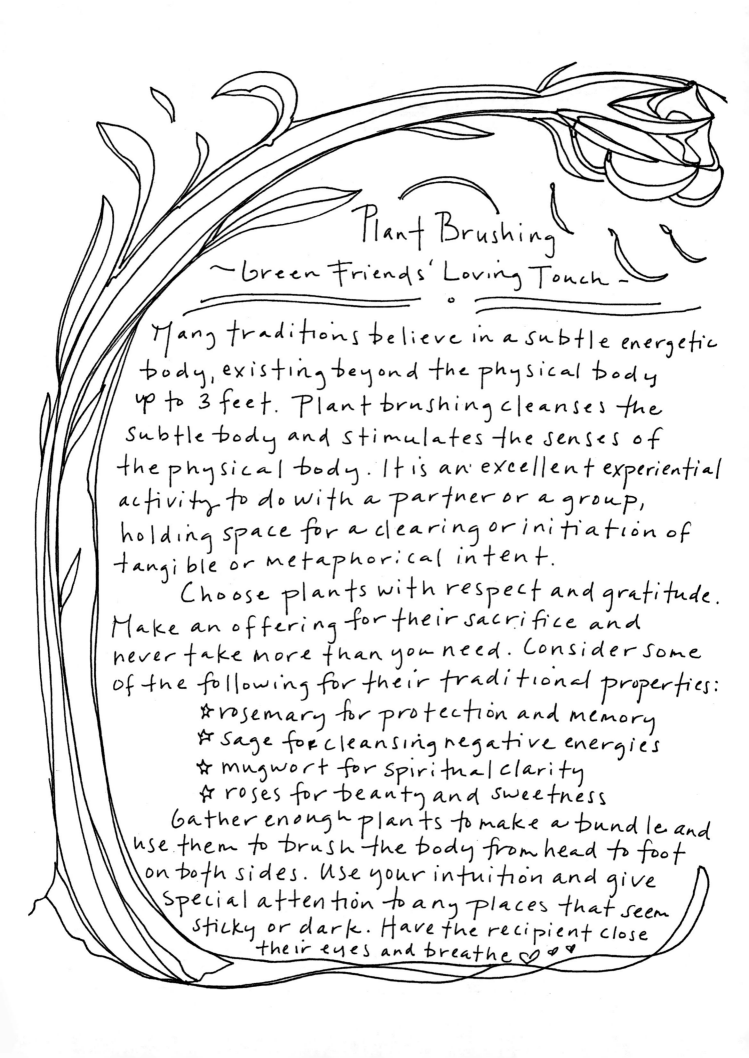

Plant Brushing
~ Green Friends' Loving Touch ~

Many traditions believe in a subtle energetic body, existing beyond the physical body up to 3 feet. Plant brushing cleanses the subtle body and stimulates the senses of the physical body. It is an excellent experiential activity to do with a partner or a group, holding space for a clearing or initiation of tangible or metaphorical intent.

Choose plants with respect and gratitude. Make an offering for their sacrifice and never take more than you need. Consider some of the following for their traditional properties:

- ✿ rosemary for protection and memory
- ✿ sage for cleansing negative energies
- ✿ mugwort for spiritual clarity
- ✿ roses for beauty and sweetness

Gather enough plants to make a bundle and use them to brush the body from head to foot on both sides. Use your intuition and give special attention to any places that seem sticky or dark. Have the recipient close their eyes and breathe ♡ ♡ ♡

...→FLOWER ESSENCES←...

Plants, too, have a subtle energetic field. The alchemy of the elements in plants creates a bioavailable mechanism for nutrients (food) to transfer to our bodies. Similarly, the essences, or energetic properties of plants, - a result of the same elemental alchemy - may be collected in a simple intentional process using springwater and sun or moonlight and preserved for use in healing. Bach flower essences are popular and available for purchase at most health and wellness stores. But homemade essences from local plants are equally viable... AND...

...homemade essences make use of your local plant friends in relationship, deepening your bioregional awareness and knowledge, thus your capacity for self-healing. Plus, the process of making your own essences is so incredibly beautiful, you won't want to miss out again. ♡♡♡

Flower and plant essences are effective for many kinds of emotional · psychological and spiritual issues. Research on correspondences is useful, but experimenting with your own intuitive experience with the plants has tremendous value. No one knows exactly "why" essences work, but determining <u>how</u> they work for you is a wonderful journey.

PREPARATIONS

You will need:
- a clear glass bowl with no ridges, markings or designs - check the bottom too!
- clean yummy water - springwater is wonderful but any will do if filtered
- flowers or plants of your choice ~ see the "choosing plants" section for harvesting & selection options
- brandy for preservation (you may use apple cider vinegar, too, if alcohol is objectionable)
- glass eyedropper bottles with glass droppers cleaned & dry
- a clear sunny day, earth to set the bowl on and several hours - see note on next page for moon essences!

1. Assemble your tools, locate your space, see what flowers wish to play. If you gather plants, make an offering, say a prayer, ask permission and stay present. You may choose to cut plants or gently blend them with the water, weighting them.

2. Rest, be easeful while the sun works its magic.

3. Remove flowers carefully after around three hours. Give thanks as you return them to the earth. Filter the water into a clean glass jar (large). Some like to leave a few petals in the essence. Take dropper bottles and fill halfway with brandy or vinegar. Top with essence, label and date. This is the mother essence. See administration and dosage on the next page. ♡ ♡♡

Some Common Correspondences for Flower Essences

from my bedside table...

Aspen : vague anxiety

Dandelion : initiative, persistence, support

Dahlia : self love

Mustard : depression and "low" feeling for no reason

Dill Flower : production

Golden Puff : Mother of Dreams

Impatiens : impatience

Quaking Aspen : opening the heart amid fear

Artichoke Heart : beauty in presence and passing

Yarrow : protection from negative influences

(based on Moon Divas and Bach)

· · ·Moon Divas Essences Portray indication by needed quality · · ·
· · ·Bach Essences indicate by deficiency · · ·

A Note on Stars Moons and Stones

Essences may be made by moonlight or starlight too! I like to infuse full moon essences for 1-2 nights prior to the full moon, which in my area means finding a platform out of critter reach. Locations can change the nature of the essence, as can the content of the water (minerals, pollutants) and the growing conditions of the plants. Your intent is also a variable. It is best to work when you feel open, centered and joyful in the process. ♡ ♡♡ (ctd...)

· · · ·ᵒUSING♡ESSENCES· · · ·

The Mother Essence should be diluted for use in glass dropper bottles filled with alcohol or 50/50 alcohol and spring water. Add essence intuitively ~ 7-10 drops is usual, but less or more may be required. Experiment. What works best for you? Working with an essence is about feeling, allowing for other ways of knowing to emerge. I select my essence allies by feeling, use 3-6 drops under my tongue a few times daily, and change essences every few weeks. Sometimes Deva and I work essences together to see what is present.

stones notes ctd ···

You may also make essences from stones or crystals ~ so fun! Though, I think the vibration of energy in stones is more sensitive to interferance, and not as easily remedied as flower work. The stones can be an excellent compliment to the essences. If you have a natural affinity for stones, this work has the same kind of intuitive promise. Try preparing a stone essence on the stone's home turf (agate essence from Agate Beach, for example). The stones contain histories much older than we can imagine. ♡ ♡ ♡

your essence notes go in the space below ↵

SPRING MENU

for detoxification, toning and building heat

First Course (starter): Wild Green Salad or Saute Dandelion, Young Nettle Tops and Chickweed are all lovely this time of year. If you are unsure about the safety of collecting greens, your local co-op or natural foods store may be able to help.

for Salad : fresh flowering Chickweed (not seedy)
fresh dandelion greens & flowers

Combine and toss with greens
- 2 cloves garlic, minced
- 2 Tbsp olive oil
- 1 Tbsp balsamic vinegar
- pinch salt & pepper
- toasted nut of choice

for Sauté : lots of dandelion greens and fresh young nettle tops*

heat together on stove
- 2 cloves garlic, chopped
- 3 Tbsp. olive oil

add to olive oil and garlic, sauté until vinegar has reduced (smells less vinegary)
- 2 Tbsp. Balsamic vinegar
- 1 Tbsp. soy sauce or Braggs
- 2 tsp Marjoram

juice of ½ lemon
chili flakes

Add greens to liquid and sauté until wilted well. Squeeze lemon over and serve hot with chili flakes.

*use caution: do not touch nettles with bare hands!

Red Coconut Curry with Jasmine Rice

warming and gently stimulating, a perfect food for cool spring days

CURRY

- 2 yams, diced
- 1 large broccoli head, cut bite-sized
- 1 red pepper, sliced
- 3 carrots, sliced
- 1 small bunch kale or new garden greens, sliced
- 1 onion, chopped
- fresh basil or cilantro, as garnish or to taste
- 2 cans coconut milk
- 3 Tbsp Thai red curry paste
- 1 Tbsp coconut oil

- Steam yams, broccoli & carrots (separately) and set aside.
- Saute onion in large pot with coconut oil until translucent.
- Add coconut milk and curry paste. Dissolve paste in milk.
- Add steamed veggies, red peppers and greens. Cook 15-20 mins.

RICE

In a large saucepan over med-low heat add:

- 3 c. water
- 1½ c. jasmine rice
- ¼ tsp salt

Turn up heat, bring water to boil then reduce to simmer and cover. Watch closely (15-20 mins) and remove from heat when all water is absorbed.

Serve curry hot over rice with basil /or /cilantro garnish. Salt to taste.

Other yummy options:
- toasted cashews
- toasted coconut
- sesame seeds

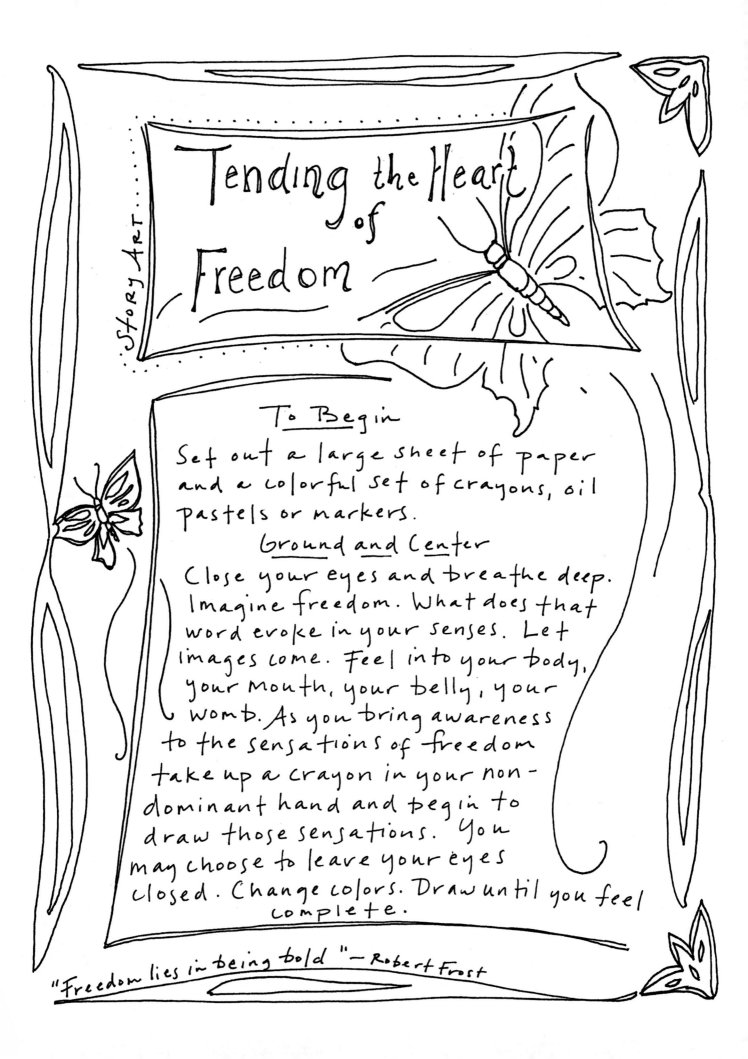

Story Art

Tending the Heart of Freedom

To Begin

Set out a large sheet of paper and a colorful set of crayons, oil pastels or markers.

Ground and Center

Close your eyes and breathe deep. Imagine freedom. What does that word evoke in your senses. Let images come. Feel into your body, your mouth, your belly, your womb. As you bring awareness to the sensations of freedom take up a crayon in your non-dominant hand and begin to draw those sensations. You may choose to leave your eyes closed. Change colors. Draw until you feel complete.

"Freedom lies in being bold" — Robert Frost

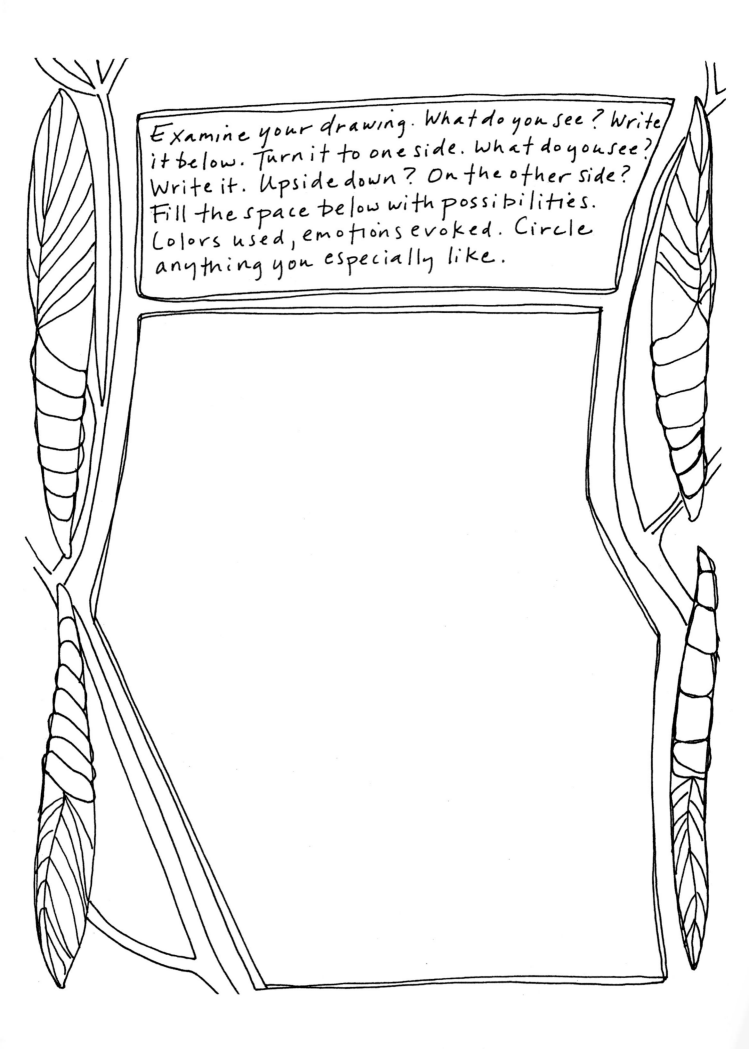

Examine your drawing. What do you see? Write
it below. Turn it to one side. What do you see?
Write it. Upside down? On the other side?
Fill the space below with possibilities.
Colors used, emotions evoked. Circle
anything you especially like.

In the space below, use your art observations to make a story. Relax and experiment. See what comes.

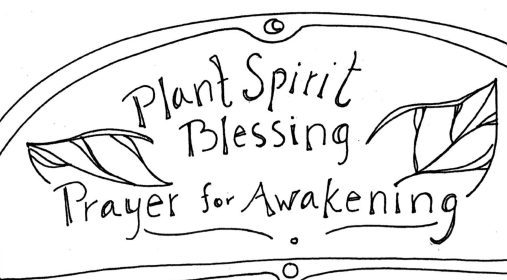

Plant Spirit Blessing
Prayer for Awakening

Dear One, Holy One
I thank you
Your breath becomes
my breath
My breath becomes
your breath
Your cells become
my cells
My cells will, in time
become
your cells.
Dear One, Holy One
I offer my gratitude
and love
That we who are so
related
May spend this day
together
Please help remember
the gifts we
share.

As we breathe
we are alive.
Good morning earth
we are alive
Winter has passed
we are alive
The root stirs
we are alive
The leaf buds
we are alive
The flower blooms
we are alive
The seed cracks
we are alive
The birds return
we are alive
The fish return
we are alive
The animals awake
I awake
I am glad to be alive

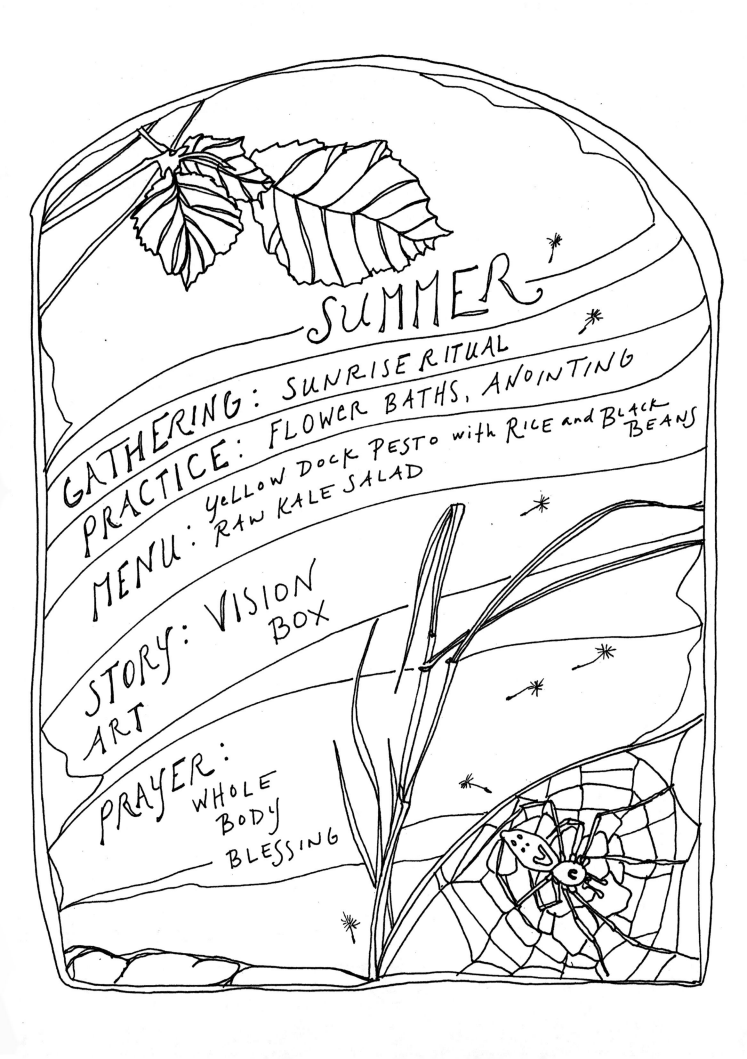

SUMMER

GATHERING: SUNRISE RITUAL

PRACTICE: FLOWER BATHS, ANOINTING

MENU: Yellow Dock Pesto with Rice and Black Beans
Raw Kale Salad

STORY: VISION BOX
ART

PRAYER: WHOLE BODY BLESSING

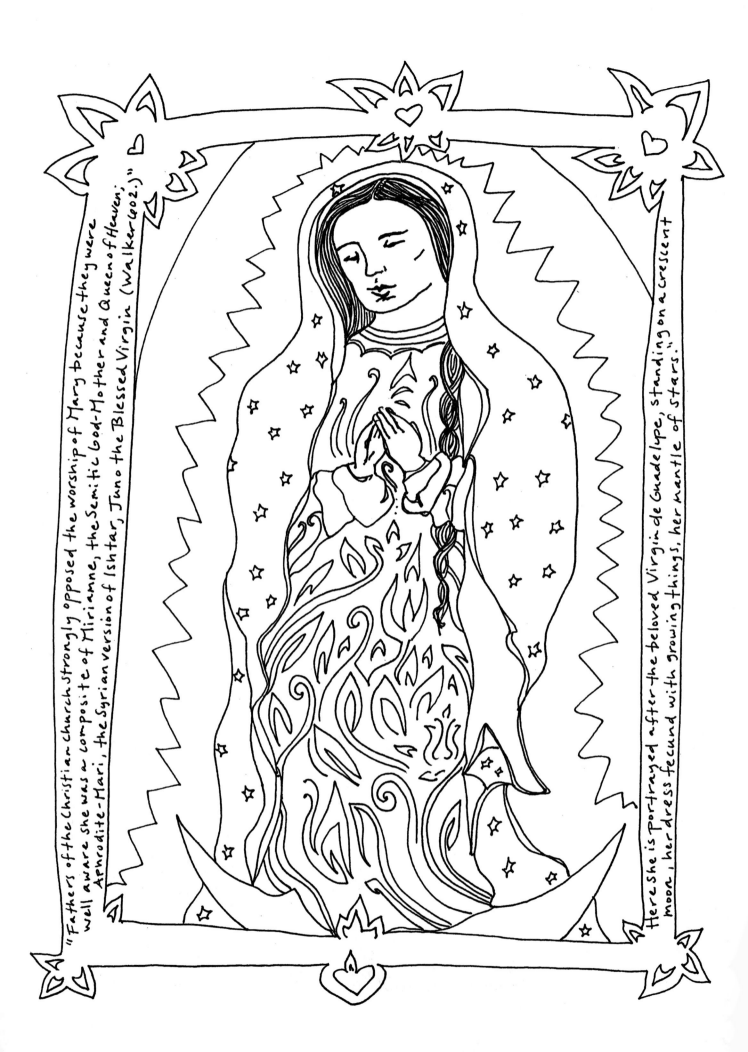

"Fathers of the Christian church strongly opposed the worship of Mary because they were well aware she was a composite of Miriamne, the Semitic God-Mother and Queen of Heaven; Aphrodite-Mari, the Syrian version of Ishtar, Juno the Blessed Virgin (Walker 402.)"

"Here she is portrayed after the beloved Virgin de Guadelupe, standing on a crescent moon, her dress fecund with growing things, her mantle of stars."

JOY and GRATITUDE

Tending the ♡ of Light in Summer

Early days and late-lit nights, summer invites activity, motion. A daily pause, to connect (bare skin to earth, water, air and sun), to reflect on the beauty and bounty of such a season, allows for the preservation (maybe literal: berry jam or peaches for winter's depth) of warmth and light within. We store the season in pantry and memory with blessings and praise.

CIRCLE SUGGESTIONS for SUMMER

☆ sunrise ritual hikes (see next page)

☆ water pilgrimages for bathing in natural waterways (river, lake, sea, spring) at the moon change

☆ first harvest blessing and meal with food from gardens or local markets or farms

☆ rituals of connection and commitment: community blessings, partnership honoring

☆ summer solstice drum and rattle rhythm night - no experience required - just bring a noisemaker and gather around the fire

☆ flower bath circle

DRINK IN BEAUTY: Hydrate in summer with herb or floral water. To one quart cold water add 3-5 newly opening roses and/or 3-5 sprigs mint (or fennel, or lavender). Refrigerate 4-6 hours and drink! Refill the jar as needed. If refrigerated herbs keep for days!

REST IN BEAUTY: Afternoon siestas are wonderfully invigorating, especially on hot days. Keep the flowers and herbs from your beauty water (above) and apply them whole and chilled to your eyes, temples and pulse points after your rest. Children of all ages love this awakening!

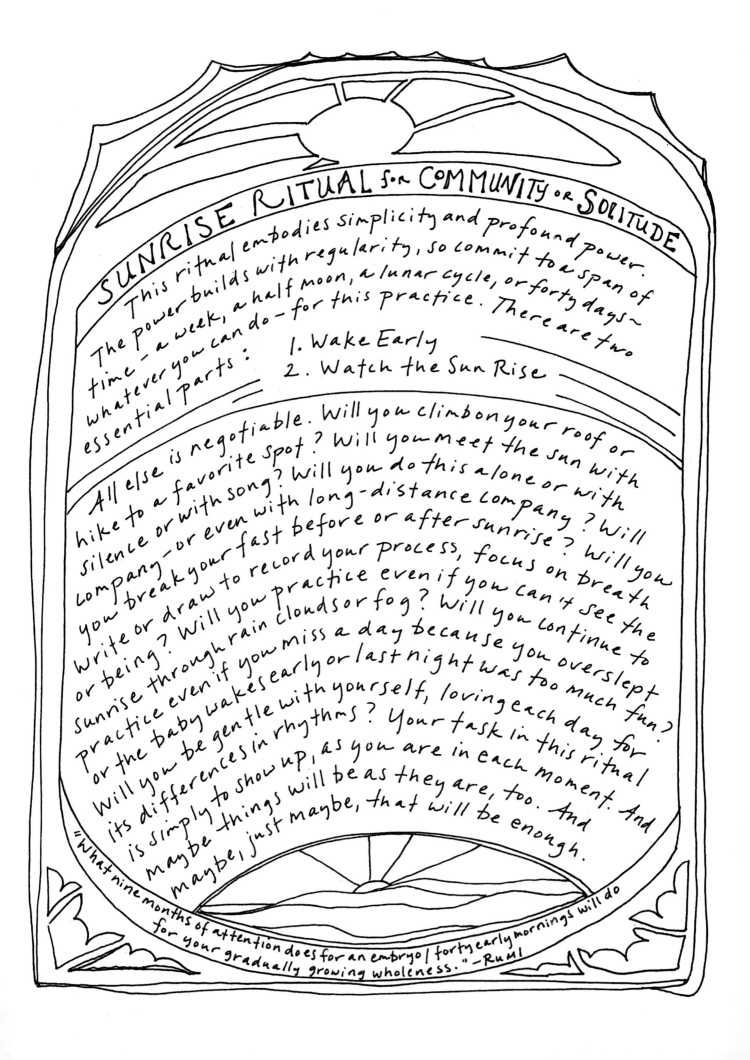

SUNRISE RITUAL for COMMUNITY or SOLITUDE

This ritual embodies simplicity and profound power. The power builds with regularity, so commit to a span of time — a week, a half moon, a lunar cycle, or forty days — whatever you can do — for this practice. There are two essential parts:

1. Wake Early
2. Watch the Sun Rise

All else is negotiable. Will you climb on your roof or hike to a favorite spot? Will you meet the sun with silence or with song? Will you do this alone or with company — or even with long-distance company? Will you break your fast before or after sunrise? Will you write or draw to record your process, focus on breath or being? Will you practice even if you can't see the sunrise through rain clouds or fog? Will you continue to practice even if you miss a day because you overslept or the baby wakes early or last night was too much fun? Will you be gentle with yourself, loving each day for its differences in rhythms? Your task in this ritual is simply to show up, as you are in each moment. And maybe things will be as they are, too. And maybe, just maybe, that will be enough.

"What nine months of attention does for an embryo / forty early mornings will do for your gradually growing wholeness." — Rumi

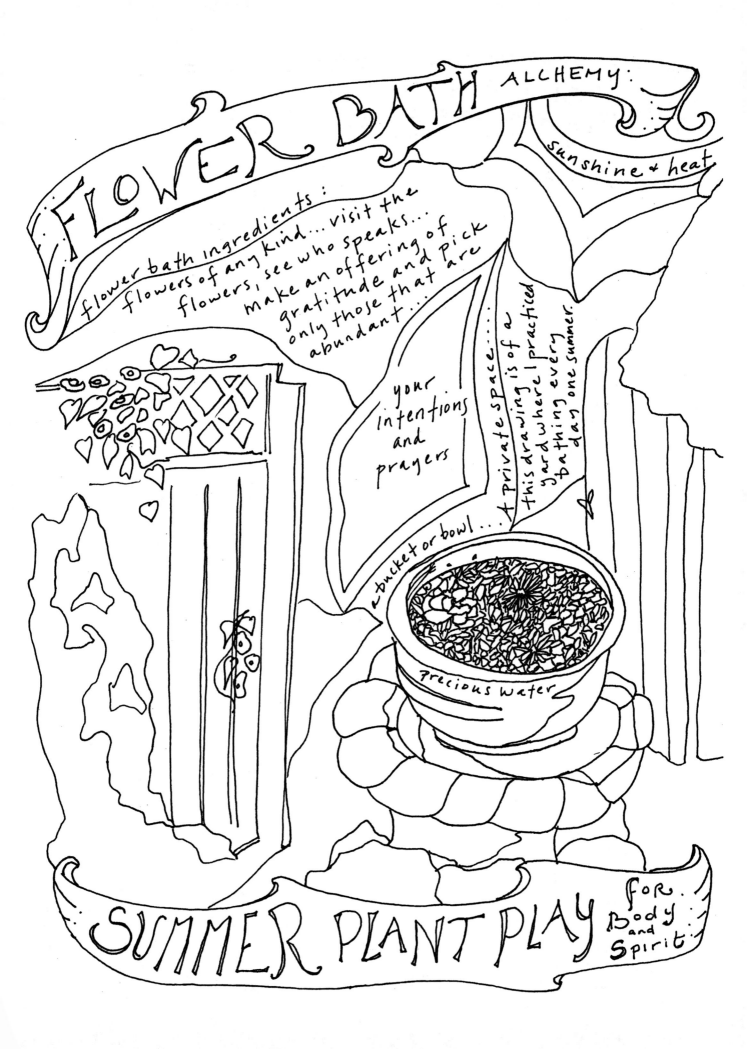

for BEAUTIFUL BATHING

Flower baths cleanse and refresh the physical and energetic body. The results are amazing! A vibrant clearing and restoration of harmonious beauty. In workshops we joke about taking before and after photos because everyone looks radiant after bathing!

You may wish to set your water out the night before your bath to infuse it with moon and starlight (and to allow any chlorine to evaporate). Bless your water. Imagine its source and journey to reach you. Bless the journey and offer thanks for this amazing and essential element.

On the morning of your bath gather flowers and aromatic leaves with respect and joy. Take pleasure in their beauty. Who are you drawn to? Ask permission. How do the flowers answer you? Leave an offering and a prayer of gratitude.

Place your flowers in your bath. Immerse your hands in the water. Set your intentions. These may be words or images, a meditation or simply a feeling. Then break the flowers and leaves into small pieces and leave the flower water to steep in the sun.

After a few hours gather a towel (for lying in the sun post-bathing) and any implements for prayers. Take a few breaths and set the space for your bath. Then disrobe to your comfort level. Scoop the bath water in your hands and throw it into the air. Let it fall all around you. Notice! Repeat! Repeat until there is enough water left to douse your head. Douse! Lie in the sun, on the earth, to dry.

MODIFICATIONS AND EXPERIMENTS

Flower baths are a remarkable seasonal practice. For those with mobility issues or those interested in developing this practice with friends, children or groups, community bathing is lovely. In community bathing a chair is used, along with a cup or shell for better control of the bath water. You may also use plant bundles or whole flowers (roses are amazing!) to sprinkle and brush bath water. It is a special treat to make a bath for a dear friend or loved one. When my daughter returns from her father's house I love to have a bath waiting for her to ease her ⟶ transition home.

ON NUDITY AND ANOINTING

The more we love and accept our bodies as they are, the more in love we can be with our bodies in the world. Nudity is a delicious freedom when we aren't worried about anyone "seeing" us or what others think. It is important to respect our comfort levels, but to not be afraid to push and question them as well. I learned to deeply love my physical body through daily flower baths in the nude. The heat of sun and air on skin, water drying in wind, tiny flecks of petals on my stretch marks and scars. I realized I had rarely seen my body whole, outside, as a woman.

To further this ritual of self love I began anointing my skin with a fragrant oil — sweet almond with rose essential oil — when I was dry, and massaging myself with a tenderness I usually reserved for others. This was at the height of my transition and this love, this gentle care began a beautiful, powerful transformation.

SUMMERTIME MENU

RINSE AND SOAK:

2 c. brown rice
(soak in cold water 1-2 hours)

2 c. black beans
(soak in cold water overnight,
refrigerate if night is warm)
be sure both dry beans and
rice are free of chaff or
stones...
♡ Drain & use soaking
water for plants...♡

then COOK

- RICE: Boil 4 c. water in
lidded saucepan. Add rice,
reduce heat and simmer
until water is absorbed
(30-45 minutes)

- BEANS: Boil 8 c. water
in large pot. Add beans,
reduce heat and simmer
until very tender, 1-2 hrs.
Add water as necessary.
When tender add vegetable
mix below.

BEAN SEASONING

- 1 yellow onion, chopped
2 carrots, chopped
1 rib celery, chopped
4 cloves garlic, minced
1 tsp chili powder
1 tsp cumin
12 oz chopped tomatoes
(1 can, or 2 fresh)
2 Tbsp soy sauce or Braggs

Sauté onions until soft, add
other vegetables and spices
with tomatoes and Braggs.
Simmer for 30 mins. Add
salt and pepper as desired.

Yellow Dock Pesto

3-4 c. greens (yellow
dock, dandelion mixed
with culinaries like basil
or oregano)
3-4 garlic cloves
1/4 c. olive oil
1/2 c. nuts (walnuts or pine
nuts or sunflower seeds)
1/4 c. parmesean cheese or
2 Tbsp. nutritional yeast

Blanch greens by covering with
water in a saucepan, bringing to
a boil and draining. Blend
greens and other ingredients
in blender or food processor until
smooth. Add salt to taste.

☆ see note on yellow dock next page

RAW KALE SALAD

1 large bunch fresh kale
2 Tbsp olive oil
2 cloves garlic, chopped
½ tsp salt

Remove stems from kale and tear into bite-sized pieces. Add olive oil and <u>Massage</u> into each piece. Take your time. The greens should soften. Then add garlic and salt and let sit (refrigerate in warm weather) an hour or two. Serve with joy!

*Thank you Shawn!

RUMEX CRISPUS   YELLOW DOCK

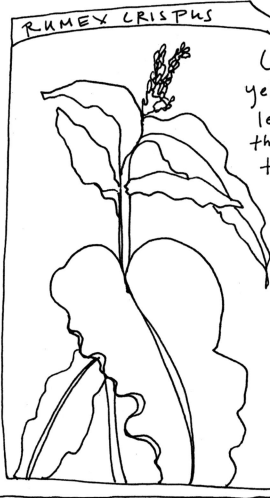

Common wayside and garden "weed," yellow dock is nutrient rich. Young leaves may be eaten in spring salads, the larger leaves must be blanched to release some bitterness. Leaves and roots are both high in iron... roots are best harvested in the fall. The abundant ruddy brown seeds grow in long clusters and have a nutty taste. I like to chew them in late summer on walks. Yellow dock is also an amazing pain reliever for insect stings, itchy bites or plant irritation. Bruise or rip a fresh leaf, mix with a bit of water (or spit) and apply directly!

Story Art:

✧ VISION BOX ✧
✧ create · believe · release ✧
✧ receive ✧

. . . Vision boxes use image art to create a 'container' for your dreams, hopes, wishes and desires. The practice of using the vision box allows for the release of our vision, creating space for it to manifest.

✧ A box of paper or wood - old recipe, stationary or cigar boxes work well
✧ magazines, catalogs, books, photos for image collection
✧ Sharp scissors
✧ a paintbrush or sponge
✧ non-toxic decoupage glue (Modge Podge) or thin white glue with water in equal parts
✧ time and space to suit your mood

YOU MAY NEED...

SAMPLE BOX
I made this box for my mother...

... the interior is collaged as well. I loved offering her a place for dreams.

♡ CREATING YOUR BOX ♡

Light a candle or set your work space in some way. Begin with selecting images - or, rather, let images select you. What and where your dreams reflect will come if you allow some space. Cut and arrange images on your box, gluing as you go, smoothing edges and bubbles. When you feel the box is complete, paint a layer of glue over the box and allow to dry overnight.

USING YOUR BOX

Articulate your vision. Make a list. Prioritize. What will serve the highest good for you and for the world?
♡ Write your first priority on a slip of paper or cloth. As you write, see the vision as if it is.

♡ As you place your first priority in the box, make an offering - incense, a prayer. Then leave the vision. Trust all is happening exactly as it needs to.
♡ You may add to your box whenever you wish. Prayers for others and blessings are lovely additions.

♡ You may empty the box whenever you desire.
♡ Cleanse the old visions by burning or burying them. Cleanse the box with sunshine or smoke.
♡ Keep a record in your journal, if you wish, of any outcomes or surprises.

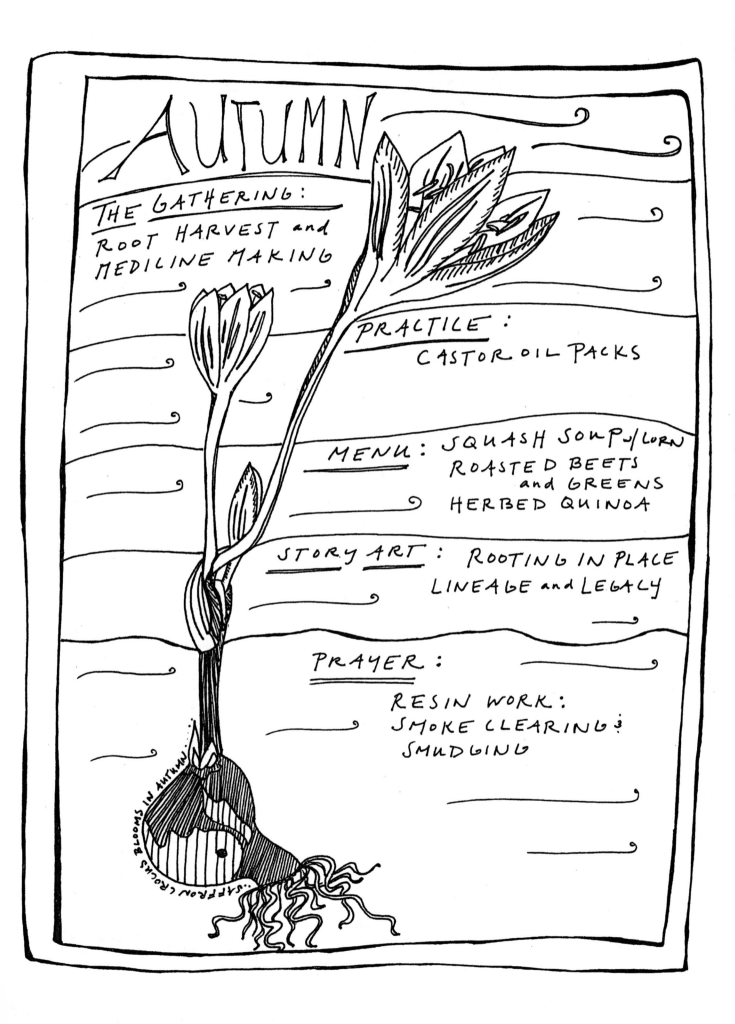

AUTUMN

THE GATHERING:
ROOT HARVEST and MEDICINE MAKING

PRACTICE:
CASTOR OIL PACKS

MENU: SQUASH SOUP w/CORN
ROASTED BEETS
and GREENS
HERBED QUINOA

STORY ART: ROOTING IN PLACE
LINEAGE and LEGACY

PRAYER:

RESIN WORK:
SMOKE CLEARING &
SMUDGING

...SAFFRON CROCUS BLOOMS IN AUTUMN...

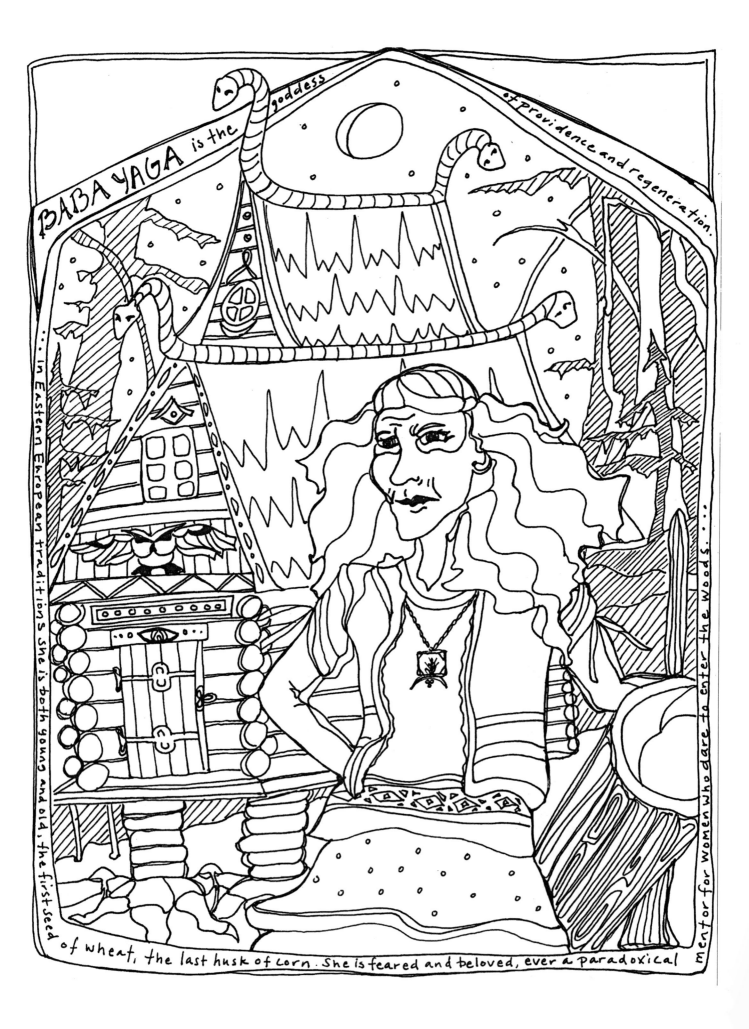

BABA YAGA is the goddess of providence and regeneration.

...In Eastern European traditions she is both young and old, the first seed of wheat, the last husk of corn. She is feared and beloved, ever a paradoxical mentor for women who dare to enter the woods...

GATHERING IN GRATITUDE AND PREPARATION

The light shifts, quality changes remind us of the shortened days. In my childhood home early autumn was a flurry of activity: pickles and preserves lining up in luminous jars, endless picking of blackberries and garden surplus for the months ahead. A tree or two cleared and cut for firewood. The work of autumn prepares us for winter, we earn our cyclical seasonal rest. Even if our lives don't require it, engaging in simple physical tasks in this time brings synchronicity and accord to our lives.

ROOTING IN ... DIGGING DEEP

In autumn, tuberous roots and taproots become richer and juicier as plant energy moves from leafy food and seed production back into the earth. Dandelions are one of my favorite fall roots to harvest, full of minerals and a whole system nourisher, Dandelion is excellent for the liver and all elimination systems. It is non-toxic and prolific, easy to identify (though be sure to distinguish between true Dandelions and certain look-alike flowers), and may be preserved and used in a number of tasty ways: roasted, pickled, fried, dried, made into apéritif.

DIG IT TOGETHER — A FALL CIRCLE SUGGESTION

Scope out the best clean (pesticide/herbicide free, not in a ditch by a road) location for your circle to dig roots. A yard is wonderful, the woods require discretion, respect and care. Above-par medicinal plants love vacant lots and open spaces... don't let the location fool you. I believe they set up shop in human territory to garner our attention. Have your circle ready to get dirty. Everyone should bring a spade or spoon, a paper bag, and if you are making vinegar or apéritif (recipes follow!) a clean dry jar. You may wish to prepare some root metaphor intentions: what are you rooting out or grounding into this season?

COMMUNITY DIG AND MAKING

If there are gardeners present they may be willing to instruct the group in the best way to dig a root while keeping (most) of the root intact (hint: go deep!). Identify a specimen of the plant you wish to gather and circle around it. You may ground in with breath, speak prayers or observations and words of gratitude to the plant. Ask for permission to dig. See what comes up. Then, slowly, dig together. Make sure everyone has a turn...

☆

As you dig, you may wish to observe silence. OR you can follow the ancient tradition of singing together as you work. The following may be set to any melody and addresses the plants directly:

⌐ Give thanks to the Earth Mother
Give thanks to the Father Sun
Give thanks to the plants before us
Where the mother and father are one.
Give thanks, Give thanks
And again I say Give thanks ⌐

After gathering the first plant, the circle may choose to gather independently the rest of the plants, or to continue together.

Dandelion Aperitif : My original experience with this medicinal

liqueur used springtime blossoms and lots of sugar. I find this autumnal blend richer and more rewarding after a full harvest meal. Chop whole dandelion plant and pack a clean dry jar. In a sauce pan dissolve 1/4 c. sugar (cane juice crystals) with good strong vodka. Pour into jar, adding more vodka until plant material is covered. Cap, label and date. Store in a cool dry place for six weeks, shaking periodically. Enjoy!

Dandelion Vinegar : in salad dressing, on greens, it's yum!

Shake the dirt off your freshly dug dandy (don't wash or wet), chop coarsely. Pack a clean dry quart jar with the whole plant and fill with apple cider vinegar. Leave some room at the top, make sure the plant is covered. Seal the jar, label and date and wait six weeks. This vinegar is wonderful for indigestion, urinary tract infections and digestive-eliminative system imbalance

aperitif additions: cardamom pods, cinnamon, lemon   Vinegar additions: garlic, chili peppers, onions ☆

AUTUMN ♡ MENU

Squash Soup with Corn

1 onion, chopped
2 cloves garlic, chopped
2 carrots, chopped
2 ribs celery, chopped
1 large or 2 smallish
  zucchini or summer
squash, sliced
2 c. corn, fresh off
  the cob (amazing!)
  or frozen
2 Tbsp. fresh basil
  chopped
1 tsp thyme
salt + pepper to taste
  2-3 c. milk or soymilk
  warmed
  1 Tbsp butter or oil

Sauté onion + garlic in oil
or butter until translucent.
Add vegetables + herbs, cover
with water or vegetable
stock + simmer until tender.
Add warm milk + salt + pepper
to taste. Serve piping hot!
♡ ♡ ♡

Roasted Beets
(with greens on! sweet!)
1 big bunch of beets ~
any color, scrubbed well +
free of dirt. Rough chop
beets + greens + place in
large roasting pan.
Drizzle with olive oil
and balsamic vinegar
(¼ c. each, or until all
is thoroughly coated)
season w/ salt + pepper +
cook, covered, in a 400°
oven until tender. Yum!
Serve with walnuts and
crumbled goat cheese.

Herbed Quinoa
1 c. quinoa (any color)
soaked at least 1 hour
and rinsed well
1 c. water
½ tsp salt
2-3 tsp chopped fresh
herbs (rosemary, oregano,
thyme, marjoram)
Boil water, add quinoa,
salt, herbs + reduce heat
to simmer, covered until
done. Watch closely,
quinoa cooks fast!
♡ ♡ ♡

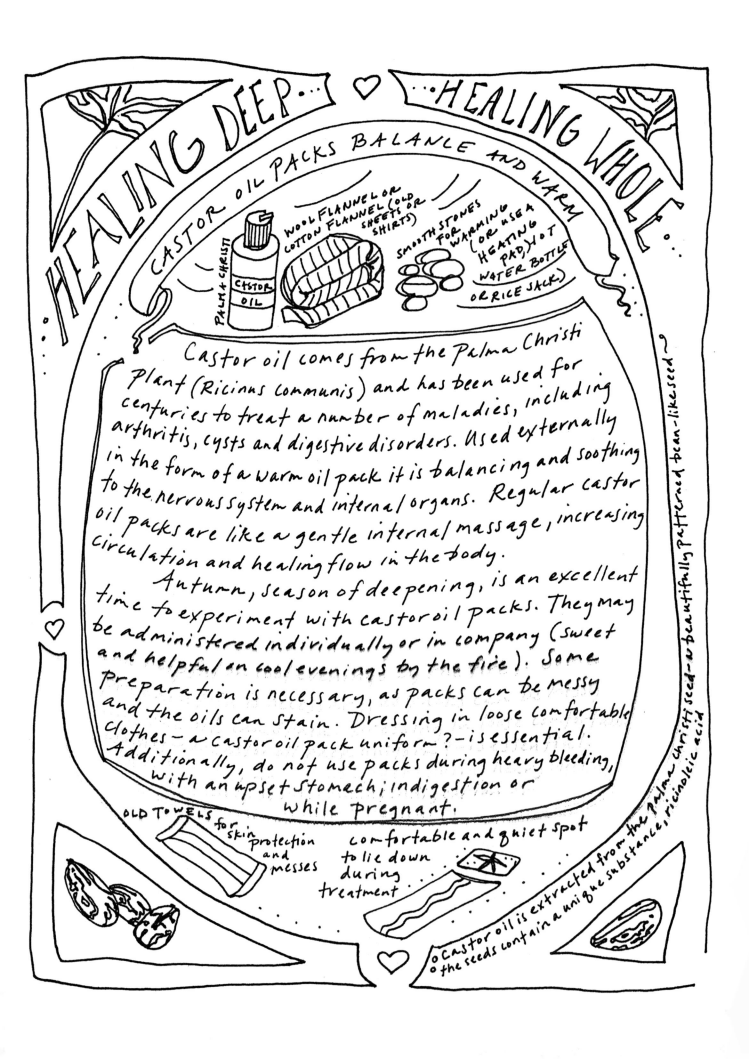

CASTOR OIL PACKS BALANCE AND WARM

PALMA CHRISTI
CASTOR OIL

WOOL FLANNEL OR COTTON FLANNEL (OLD SHEETS OR SHIRTS)

SMOOTH STONES FOR WARMING (OR USE A HEATING PAD, HOT WATER BOTTLE OR RICE SACK)

Castor oil comes from the Palma Christi plant (Ricinus communis) and has been used for centuries to treat a number of maladies, including arthritis, cysts and digestive disorders. Used externally in the form of a warm oil pack it is balancing and soothing to the nervous system and internal organs. Regular castor oil packs are like a gentle internal massage, increasing circulation and healing flow in the body.

Autumn, season of deepening, is an excellent time to experiment with castor oil packs. They may be administered individually or in company (sweet and helpful on cool evenings by the fire). Some preparation is necessary, as packs can be messy and the oils can stain. Dressing in loose comfortable clothes — a castor oil pack uniform? — is essential. Additionally, do not use packs during heavy bleeding, with an upset stomach, indigestion or while pregnant.

OLD TOWELS for skin protection and messes

comfortable and quiet spot to lie down during treatment

castor oil is extracted from the palma christi seed — a beautifully patterned bean-like seed

○ castor oil is extracted from the palma christi seed
○ the seeds contain a unique substance, ricinoleic acid

☆ BEFORE the PACK ☆ ☆

Gather your supplies. Castor oil and flannel are available at most natural foods stores. I use an old thick cotton flannel shirt cut into 12"×12" pieces for my pack and it works well. If you are using stones, place them in a crock pot with water for an hour or so before the session. Make sure you protect any carpet with an old towel. Are you in a quiet space where you won't be disturbed? Turn off the phone. Clear your calendar for the evening. This deep work can move a lot of emotions. Give yourself the gift of time and space. Set an intention for the practice. Ground and center. You may wish to light a candle, dim the house lights, breathe deeply, meditate and pray before continuing. ☆

You will be applying oil, layers of flannel cloth, towels and a heat source to your body. Where do you need healing and connection? Soothing and balance? Castor oil is wonderful for the breasts, the heart, the belly and the womb. It can be helpful to focus on one area at a time, rather than trying to do it all in one session. Listen to your body. What needs your attention? →

↓DURING☆

Pour a generous amount of castor oil into your hands. Warm it by rubbing your hands together then apply it to the place you wish to pack. Layer flannel over the oil, then a towel over the flannel. Apply your heat source. *Caution* if using hot rocks do not handle directly. Use a slotted spoon to remove them from the water and great care in placement. Cover with another towel. Make sure you are warm and comfortable. Breathe. Close your eyes and see where your breath directs you. Remain for at least 20 mins and as long as an hour. ←

☆AFTER☆

Remove the pack. Massage in any excess oil. The oil soaked flannel may be used repeatedly for treatment. Store in a plastic bag in a cool dry place.

Take time to write-draw-reflect on your experience. See what comes up. You may wish to rest or sleep after the pack. Eat light, drink lots of water and be well...

STORY ART: Where are you From?
What do you Leave Behind?

In every great story there is a plot (what's happening) and often — sometimes subtlely — a character (starring: you!) and a landscape where the tale unfolds. Modern literature — a place or setting, at times relegates place to the sidelines, and so, as it turns out, do we.

By connecting, acknowledging, building intimacy with the places we inhabit, we may begin to see how (or if) they serve us, and how we may serve them. How does your place — home, house, neighborhood, town, city, watershed, bioregion, state, country — inform your story? Does your place assist you in writing the new story you wish to live? Look deeper. What in your place does support you? If not, why? Look deeper. What in your place does nurture you? How can you root where you are? If your place is not serving your new story, or is temporary, what actions can you take to honor the place you live better and more beautiful?

"If you don't know where you are, you don't know who you are." Wendell Berry ♡

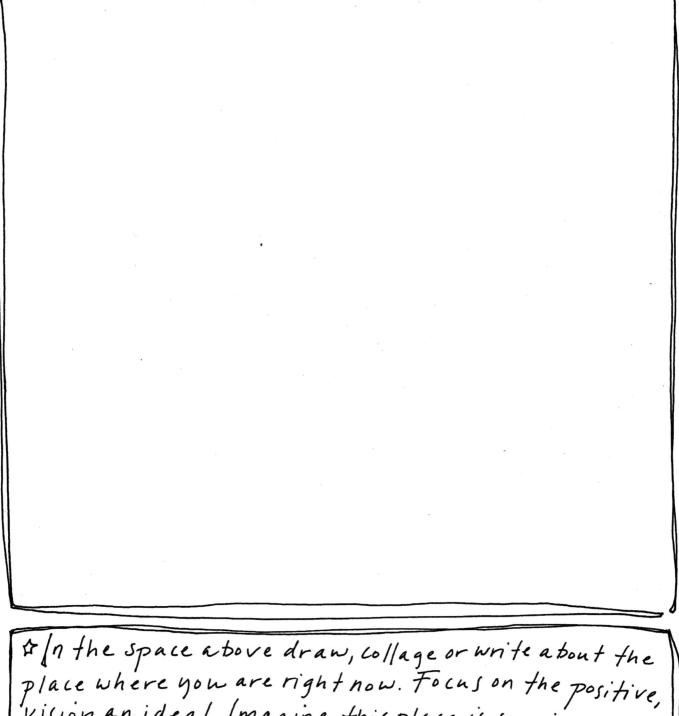

the NOW PLACE

☆ In the space above draw, collage or write about the place where you are right now. Focus on the positive, vision an ideal. Imagine this place is serving a powerful purpose in your life's journey, aiding you without cease as you discover your gifts. Play, pretend. How are you loved by where you are? What can you do to facilitate communication with this place, right now, where you are?

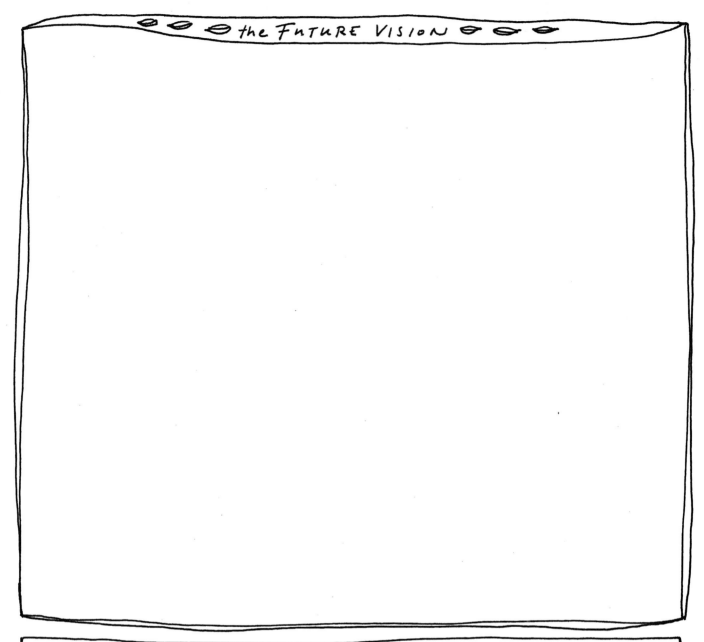

the FUTURE VISION

☆ Where do you wish to be ten years from now? In the space above, visualize your home, landscape and community. Don't try to control the words or images, let them come. Allow for surprise. Use all of your senses. Then, look for correspondences with your now place story art. What can you tend to now, through action and service, to facilitate your vision of what may be?

PRAYER
to the heavens

Smoke is an ancient offering, still present in many spiritual traditions. Smoke represents transformation—matter into ether—connection and communication with the greater, the beyond. Smoke may be used to clear and cleanse a space for ritual or practice. Incense is resin, ground and formed into sticks, though not all incense is free from chemicals. My favorite smoke is from the wood of the palo santo, or "holy wood" tree, said to take prayers to heaven and seal intentions. I also love copal resin, which may be crushed and burned on charcoal. Both of these are gifts from Deva's ventures in South America. Locally, I collect cedar and sage, dry them in tight bundles, and use them with regularity until the scent alone is enough to bring me into reverence.

Palo Santo stick burning at my desk as I write....

Smoke Offering and Prayer to the Circle

Breathe deeply and ground yourself. Notice where you are, the four cardinal directions. Bless your smoke wood, incense or resin. Bless, as you light it, your implement of fire. You may begin at any direction you choose, though this writing begins with the East. Raise your smoke to that direction. You may be silent or speak words of gratitude aloud. You may wish to investigate traditional associations with each direction, or you may wish to rely on your intuition. Both are correct. Open your heart and allow the offering to flow through you.

To the East.
To the South.
To the West.
To the North.
To the Sky - Stars - Universe Above.
To the Earth. Below.

Surround yourself with smoke. Offer gratitude to your ancestors, to all that sustains you, the miraculous, at the center of such beauty.

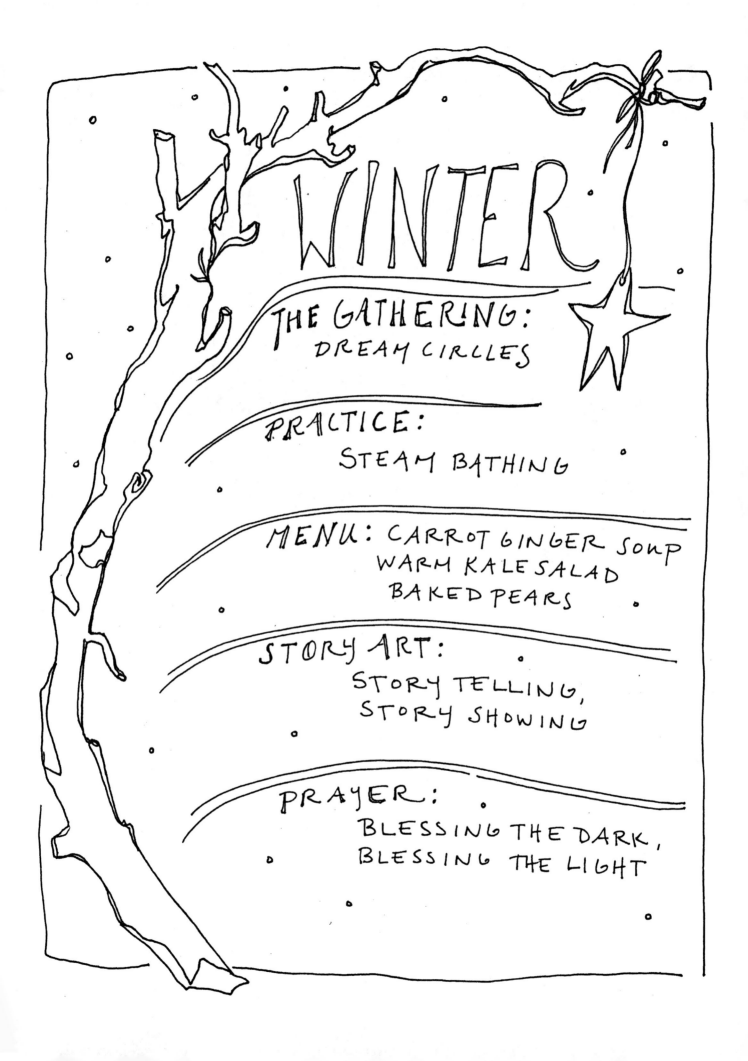

WINTER

THE GATHERING:
DREAM CIRCLES

PRACTICE:
STEAM BATHING

MENU: CARROT GINGER SOUP
WARM KALE SALAD
BAKED PEARS

STORY ART:
STORY TELLING,
STORY SHOWING

PRAYER:
BLESSING THE DARK,
BLESSING THE LIGHT

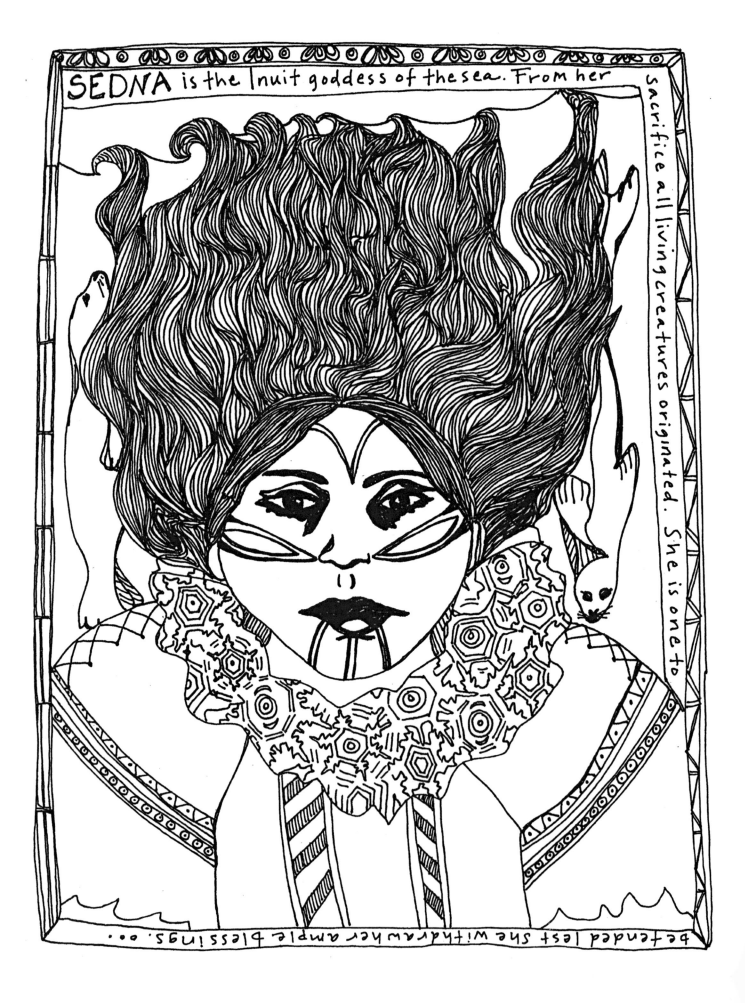

SEDNA is the Inuit goddess of the sea. From her sacrifice all living creatures originated. She is one to be defended lest she withdraw her ample blessings...

SEASONAL RHYTHM & SEASON WITHIN

I realize this book is bioregionally centered. I live in the (at times) distinctly four seasoned Pacific Northwest, marked by dark wet winters. Yet, there is, I believe, a translation of season, rhythm and tradition beyond the boundaries of my experience. Wherever we reside there is an opportunity for traditions of cycle: light and dark, activity and rest, receptivity and release. Rhythmic tradition honors life in all of its complexity and offers, in each season, something of delight, something of deepening. A reason to gather, to practice, to be present in the turning wheel and live fully in each day.

DARKNESS is for DREAMING

An ode to slumber, the winter's circle may choose to sleep over, to nest around a fire for storytelling, steam baths and setting space for long nights of collective dreams. Yes, a slumber party is suggested, with a light meal and intention setting, with a slow evening, meditations or readings, soft music, dream tea and morning gathering for revealing what the night offered to all.

Of course, there is also the possibility of delayed dreaming, late night talks and snacks, higher energy and music making. But gathering in darkness, celebrating the wonders of the still time, the shift and pulse toward solstice, the turn again to light, is the joy of wintertime.

Steam Baths

Healing heat is a conduit for the nourishment from volatile compounds from plants. Steam baths may be used on various parts of the body (face, hands and feet) but are traditionally practiced for the pelvis and vagina, where the alchemical forces of warmth, water and plants combine to prevent, soothe and treat many common difficulties.

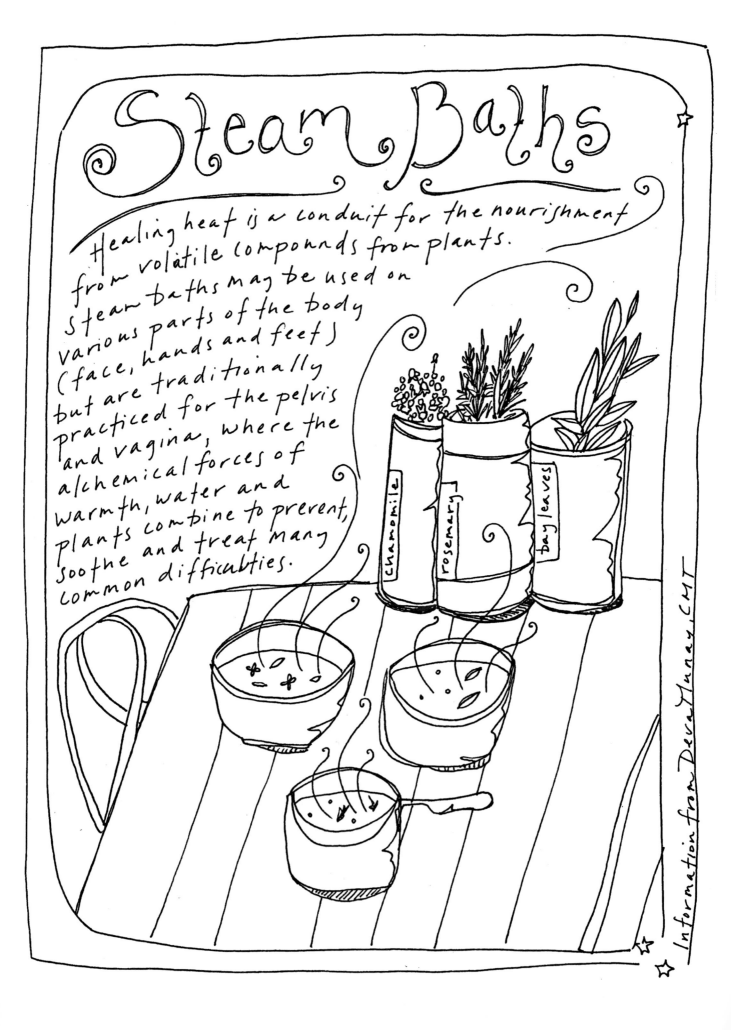

chamomile

rosemary

bay leaves

Information from Deva Munay, CMT

Cleanse your space with smoke (see Autumn) or plant brushing (see Spring). Pine, cedar and fir are all fragrant and good for clearing. You may choose to brush yourself, too.

Light a large pillar candle—one that won't tip over or burn down too quickly.

☆ As you prepare your bath, take deep breaths and feel into your body. What do you sense?

Take a moment to write or draw your preliminary sensations.

As you steam, try not to think, instead, breathe. Allow thoughts and impressions to rise. If you become distracted, focus on the breath.

After steaming, it is important to rest and integrate. In the morning, set aside some time to write or create as an exploration of what the steam brought up.

Choose a Space and Time

Free from distractions and interruptions. Night is best for relaxing after the steam and an opportunity to go deep in celebration of winter's stillness.

Turn off all electronics and phones. If you choose music, let it be consistent and relaxing.

(((STEAM)))
(((RITUAL)))

CONSIDERATIONS FOR THE RITUAL...

☆ If you don't feel ready or cannot participate in a vaginal steam, facial steams are wonderfully opening and relaxing.

☆ It may seem awkward, but facilitating a steam for another, or having a steam gifted to you is an amazing luxury. Also, steaming in community with women you trust is mind-blowing, truly transformative power.

~Preparing the Steam~

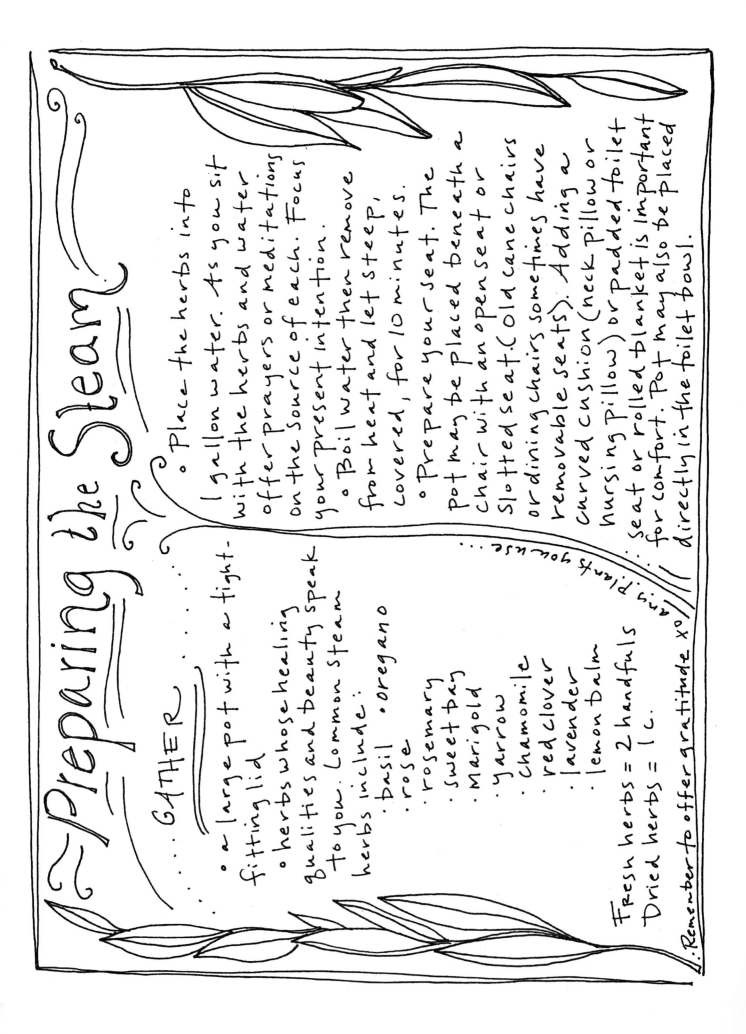

....GATHER....

- a large pot with a tight-fitting lid
- herbs whose healing qualities and beauty speak to you. Common steam herbs include:
  - Basil
  - oregano
  - rose
  - rosemary
  - sweet bay
  - Marigold
  - yarrow
  - chamomile
  - red clover
  - lavender
  - lemon balm

Fresh herbs = 2 handfuls
Dried herbs = 1 c.

- Place the herbs into 1 gallon water. As you sit with the herbs and water offer prayers or meditations on the source of each. Focus your present intention.
- Boil water then remove from heat and let steep, covered, for 10 minutes.
- Prepare your seat. The pot may be placed beneath a chair with an open seat or slotted seat. (Old cane chairs or dining chairs sometimes have removable seats). Adding a curved cushion (neck pillow or nursing pillow) or padded toilet seat or rolled blanket is important for comfort. Pot may also be placed directly in the toilet bowl.

...Or simply, air if you should...

...Remember to offer gratitude xo

• Steams are best practiced just before menstruation.

• Changes in menstrual or vaginal discharge after a steam are part of normal cleansing. However, any changes that cause pain or concern should be discussed with your medical practitioner.

○ Women trying to conceive should steam only from the first day of menstruation until ovulation.

○ Steams are not recommended for women who are pregnant. However, steams may be effective for post-partum healing.

• Steams are best in the evening, directly before bed. It is important to stay _warm_ after the steam, to lie down and allow your body to integrate the experience and attention you have provided. Quiet rest + space is an essential part of steaming.

☆

...STEAMING & DREAMING...

Remove all clothes below your waist. Keep a sweater or shawl handy for your upper body. Sit on the chair over the uncovered pot. Test the steam. It should not be burning _hot_. Cover your lower body and the chair base with a blanket. The blanket should surround you with the opening in front so you may let out heat in the beginning. Once you are comfortable, relax. Meditate. Dream. Breathe.

☆ ☆ ☆

The steam should last for around twenty minutes. Keep your upper body warm and end the steam before it gets cold. Steams are a wonderful time to connect with your womb, to visualize light and energy entering and clearing your pelvis. It is a time to deeply open and ...receive...

BAKED PEARS
with cardamom

"where those who loved you rushing back to their intimate stalls held out pears that had been dreamed for you."
— Brenda Hillman

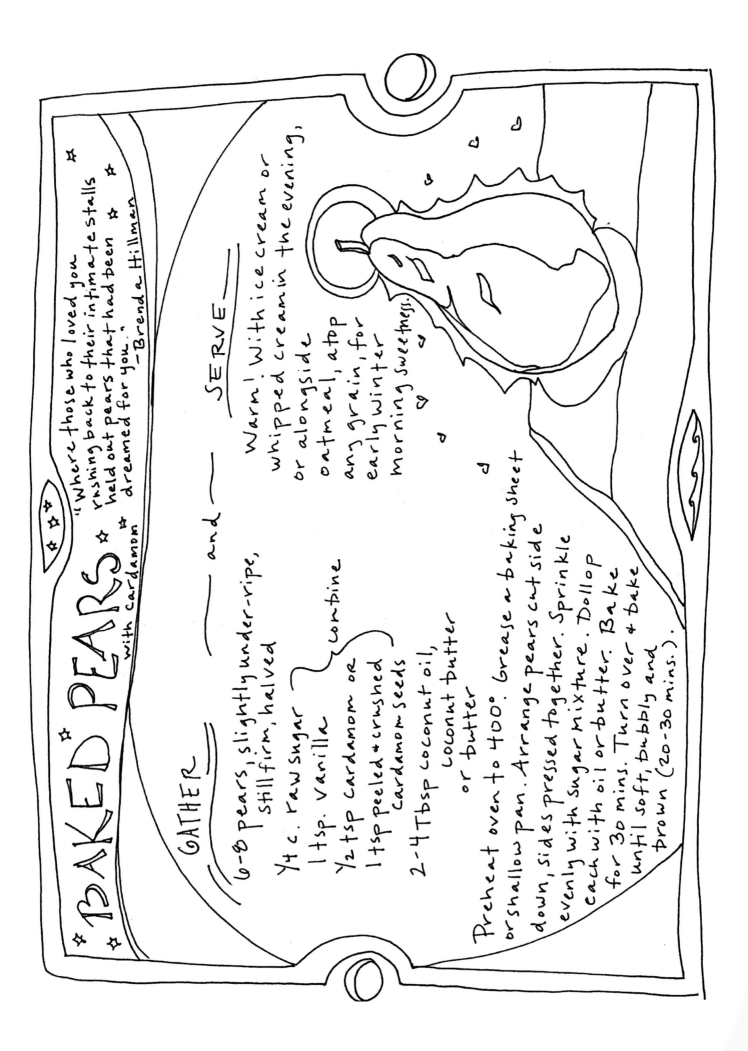

GATHER — and —

6-8 pears, slightly under-ripe, still firm, halved

¼ c. raw sugar ⎫
1 tsp. vanilla ⎬ combine
½ tsp cardamom or ⎭
1 tsp peeled + crushed
   cardamom seeds

2-4 Tbsp coconut oil,
   coconut butter
   or butter

Preheat oven to 400°. Grease a baking sheet or shallow pan. Arrange pears cut side down, sides pressed together. Sprinkle evenly with sugar mixture. Dollop each with oil or butter. Bake for 30 mins. Turn over + bake until soft, bubbly and brown (20-30 mins.).

— SERVE —

Warm! With ice cream or whipped cream in the evening, or alongside oatmeal, atop any grain, for early winter morning sweetness.

FEASTING by CANDLELIGHT

CARROT GINGER SOUP

2 lbs carrots, chopped
Place in medium-large pot, cover with water, bring to boil and simmer until tender.

In another sauce pan sauté the following:
2 T. coconut oil
2 medium onions, chopped
2 T. ginger, minced
2 tsp. mint
1 tsp. turmeric
1 tsp. cumin
1/4 tsp. coriander
1/4 tsp. cayenne
1 tsp. salt
1/2 lemon (juice)

1/4 - 1/2 c. cashews, raw or toasted, soaked

Blend cooked carrots, sauté and cashews with hand blender or in standard blender. Add water/salt as desired.

Serve piping hot with a sprinkle of toasted cashews on top.

thank you Deva!

WARM GREENS SALAD

1 large bunch winter greens (kale, chard, collards)
Wash, trim stems and chop
3 cloves garlic, chopped
2 T. olive oil
2 T. balsamic vinegar
1 T. Braggs or soy sauce
1 T. marjoram

Sauté garlic and marjoram in olive oil on medium heat for a few minutes. Add balsamic vinegar and soy sauce. Allow vinegar to reduce and thicken in the pan. Add kale and cook until soft but not mushy.

serve with

Herbed quinoa from the autumn menu, rice millet or other whole grains are a delicious compliment to these tangy greens and sweet-warm soup.

Good company, music, lit candles and the smell of baked pears (next page)... a cozy winter's meal.

Blessing the Dark

To all beings who reside in the spaces between, filament of root, depth of soil, light years to another star, I sing this gratitude. To the turning time, essential, the resting and within, the dream of what may be and grow, I sing this gratitude. To the fallow, the inward, the obscure unknown, the shape of still branches, I sing this gratitude. To what is that I cannot see, crossroads, ocean trough, beyond this living veil, to other sides, I sing this gratitude. For as the promise of death makes us living, so does the promise of winter make us spring. Holy darkness, blessed is this being and whole. Together.

Blessing the Light

To the generous burn of our only warming star, to the multitude of glints that hint at a possibility beyond our own, I sing this gratitude. To the gracious tip of earth, the waking seed, the green makers in every leaf awaiting only sun, I sing this gratitude. To the spirit that is respiration, to the processes and rhythms that create all living breath, I sing this gratitude. For each day we awaken, the promise of warmth, the gift of sight, each delicious color and texture created by the pulse and miracle of a passion greater and more beautiful than any other we can hope to know.

A Spring Amid the Ice:

STORYTELLING AS LIGHT IN THE DARK

Light the candles and circle in close and I will tell you the story of Baba Yaga... in a moment. First, may our bellies be full, may the tea be hot. May the night be long, ancient, cold and black. May the winds howl, the rain curtail our sight, for these are the nights of story gifts. Stories of our ancestors. Myths of our grandmothers. Stories of vision, adventure and courage. Stories of creativity, of futures where we wish to be. Stories we have saved to savor on the longest nights.

When we gather stories, when we take the ones we love inside through memorization or artistic recollection (read: making up parts) we honor one of our oldest human traditions. When we make the telling a ritual, gather in winter with the stories we have saved all year, we invoke a deep, abiding and joyous power. We link, past + present, old + new, each to each. We increase consciousness, _fun_, and love.

♡ ♡ ♡

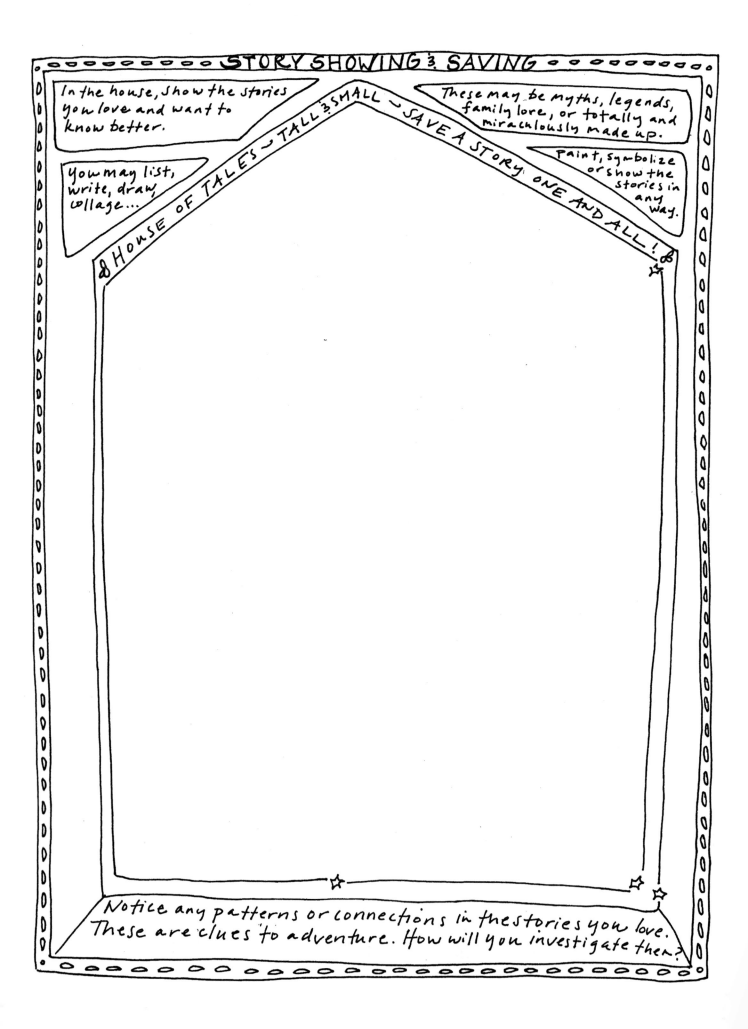

In the house, show the stories you love and want to know better.

You may list, write, draw, collage...

These may be myths, legends, family lore, or totally and miraculously made up.

Paint, symbolize or show the stories in any way.

HOUSE OF TALES ~ TALL & SMALL ~ SAVE A STORY ONE AND ALL!

Notice any patterns or connections in the stories you love. These are clues to adventure. How will you investigate them?

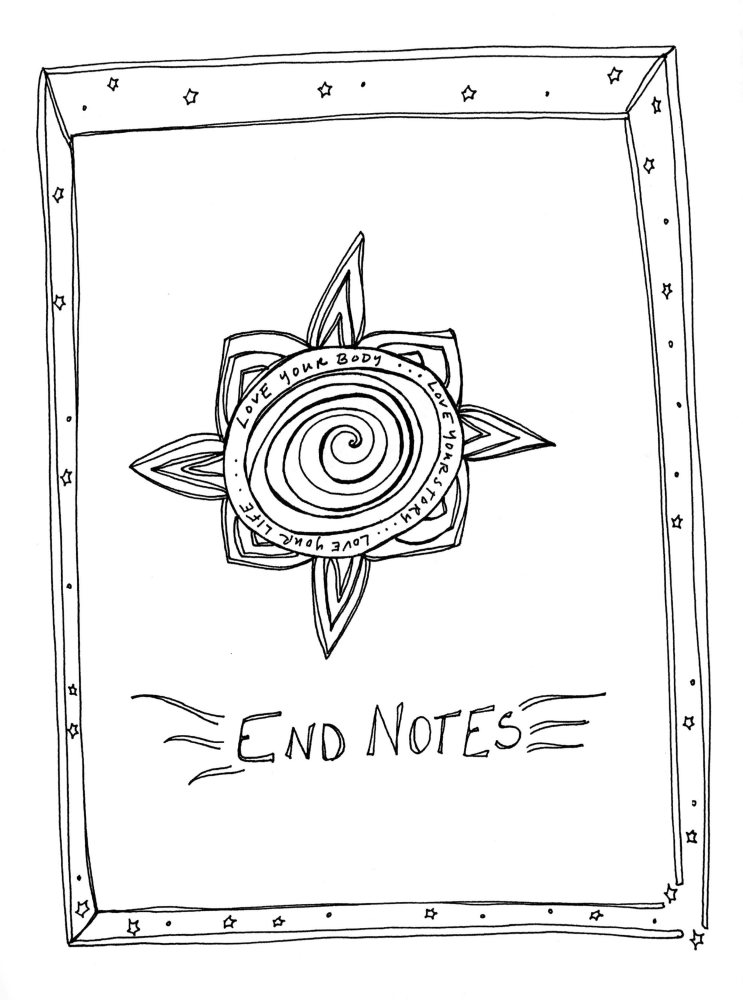

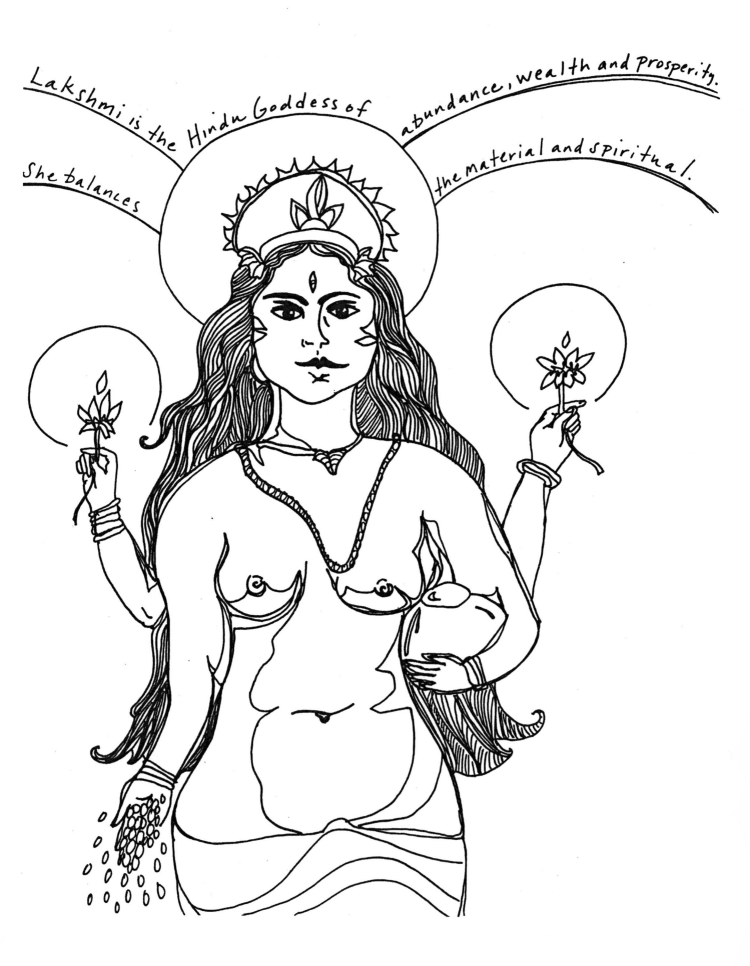

Lakshmi is the Hindu Goddess of abundance, wealth and Prosperity. She balances the material and spiritual.

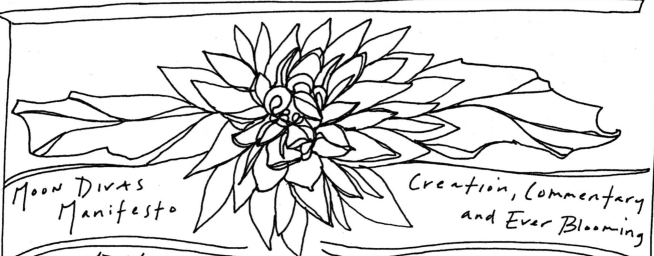

Moon Divas Manifesto

Creation, Commentary and Ever Blooming

The MD Manifesto was inspired by both our personal experiences and the expressions of our students. At the center of so many of our depressions and limitations, our stories, was a sense of inadequacy and a discomfort - or even terror - of seeing and celebrating our unique beauties. Our self-love was minimized and always conditional: dependent on the approval of others or fulfillment of some sort of social conditioning, such as losing weight.

Why was it so difficult for us to love ourselves right now, with all of our beauties and flaws? The answer to that question is long, historical, the legacy of both patriarchy and capitalism. But also in the answer is the manifesto's seed: it isn't hard for women to love themselves. It is just something most of us have never been taught to do. In community, in safety, we learn healing and connectivity - and this is self-love. We expand our personal authority with knowledge of our own bodies, our stories, women's history and myth, rites and mysteries. With practice we may unravel the threads that bind us to stories we do not wish to live. With the practice of self-care and tenderness we create new stories and model behaviors that represent a way of being and honoring all life.

For, when you live your life as an expression of love and reverence, you will see the miraculous gift each life may be, both human and non-human. All of the energy we spend feeling inadequate is meant for our calling, for serving something greater than our own reflection. Self-love is the first step to selfless service, to living a life of meaning and offering your unique gifts to the world.

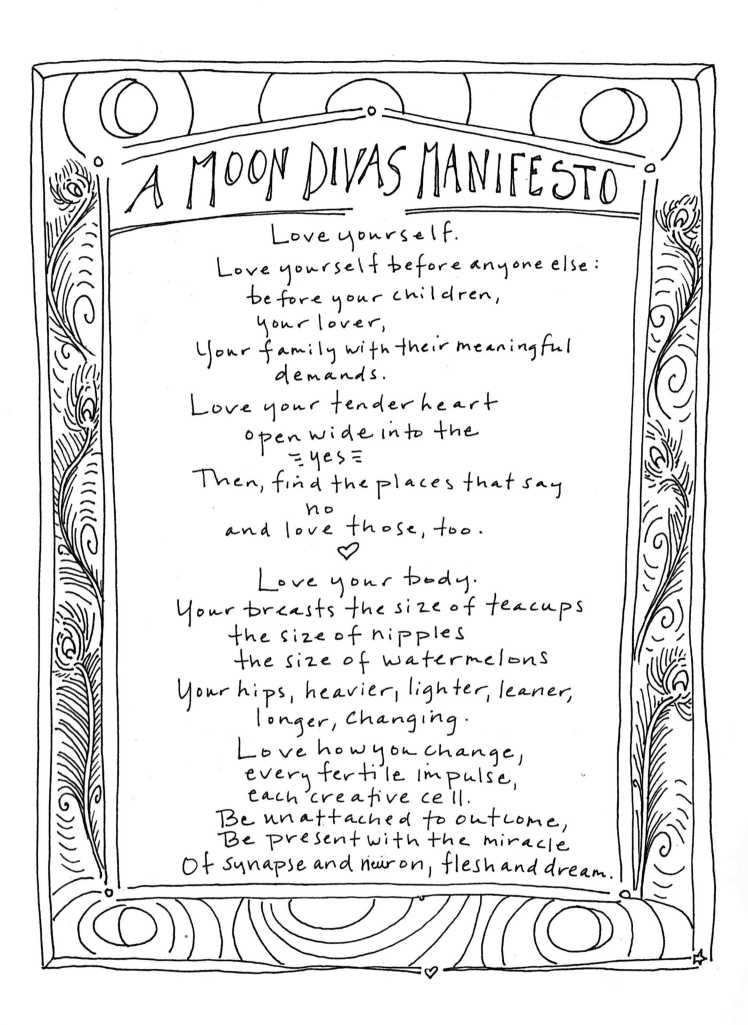

A MOON DIVAS MANIFESTO

Love yourself.
Love yourself before anyone else:
before your children,
your lover,
your family with their meaningful
demands.
Love your tender heart
open wide into the
≡ yes ≡
Then, find the places that say
no
and love those, too.
♡

Love your body.
Your breasts the size of teacups
the size of nipples
the size of watermelons
Your hips, heavier, lighter, leaner,
longer, changing.
Love how you change,
every fertile impulse,
each creative cell.
Be unattached to outcome,
Be present with the miracle
Of synapse and neuron, flesh and dream.

Love More.
More!
More than your fingernails
Or your ability to
touch your toes.
Love the way your belly ripples,
Love the stretch marks — Growth!
Rough skin — Strength!
Pimples and scars — Ours!
Love the mark that is only you:
the chipped tooth,
the curled up toe that never looks right.
= It is =
= All =
= Right. =

Love your womb,
receptor, opener,
deep place of beginning.
Place your hand on her,
the she in you.
Even if she is a spirit womb
she calls to you to Listen.
♡
Listen.
I know it seems impossible.
Our habits pattern hatred.
Voices in past stories may say "never,"
May say worse.

But, dear
ones,
Please listen:
this is the most powerful
tool that we can practice,
that we can learn and relearn
and teach
to daughters and sons,
mothers and fathers,
sisters and brothers,
An act of contrition and creation
that sets us whole:
to love ourselves in full,
That who you are, right now,
without alteration
is enough
and beauty
enough and more.
You are everything
divine and holy
Your life connected and
expressing all
the wonders of nature and
creation.
You are a sacred gift,
worthy of your own love.
We all are.

Brightest blessings and most Holy Grace to my dear spirit-sister and partner in this sweet endeavor, Ms. Deva Munay. Without your wisdom, moxie, ceremony, joy and verve, this book would not be. Your creations and contributions are essential to the whole and I honor you as one of my greatest teachers. You inspire me to move, speak, play and stretch my edges. Thank you. Amazing woman, I love you always.

This book is our work, Moon Divas a synthesis of our unique abilities. Though mostly created while you were in Peru, your presence was felt through the entire process.

HONORING THE TEACHERS, BLESSING THE PROCESS

The information in this book is one of lineage, a great tradition spanning time & cultures too numerous to name. Deva and I have benefited from the work of many teachers in this tradition, including - but never limited to - the following: Merlin Stone, Starhawk, Marija Gimbutas, Vicki Noble, Clarissa Pinkola Estés, Barbara Walker, Diane Stein, Riane Eisler, Sue Monk Kidd, Louise Erdrich, Keri Smith, Rosemary Gladstar, Susun Weed, Margot Adler, Shekhinah Mountainwater, Ffiona Morgan, Eve Ensler, Ina May Gaskin, Sharon Doubiago. Terry Tempest Williams, Sobonfu Somé, Sister Spirit, We'Moon, and so many more... Deva would particularly like to honor Rosita Arvigo and her work with Nadine Epstein in the books Spiritual Bathing: Healing Rituals and Traditions from Around the World, and Rainforest Home Remedies: The Maya Way to Heal Your Body and Replenish Your Soul. May this work of ours be an offering, a praise to our teachers and the Divine.

☆ WORKS CITED OR CONSULTED ☆

Atlas of Human Anatomy. Surrey, UK : Taj Books LTD, 2009.

Eiker, Diane and Sapphire, Eds. Keep Simple Ceremonies. Portland, Maine : Astarte White Shell Press, 1993.

Munay, Deva. "Self-Care Worksheets." Boulder, CO, 2008-10.

Northrup, Christiane. Women's Bodies, Women's Wisdom. New York : Bantam, 1994.

Stein, Diane. All Women are Healers. Freedom, CA : The Crossing Press, 1990.

Telesco, Patricia. 365 Goddess. NY : Harper Collins, 1998.

Walker, Barbara G. The Woman's Encyclopedia of Myths and Secrets. New York : Harper Collins, 1983.

Weed, Susun. Healing Wise. Woodstock, NY : Ash Tree Publishing, 1989.

A note on format: the choice to handwrite this book was inspired by authors such as Keri Smith (How to Be an Explorer of the World), Alicia Bay Laurel (Living on the Earth) and Raleigh Briggs (Make Your Place), all unique and inspirational books.

☆ TEXTS MENTIONED / RECOMMENDED ☆

Abrams, Rachel Carlton, MD, and Chia Mantak. The Multi-Orgasmic Woman. New York : Rodale, 2005.

Ensler, Eve. The Vagina Monologues. New York : Villard Books, 1998.

Kent, Tami Lynn. Wild Feminine. Hillsboro, OR : Beyond Words, 2011.

Muscio, Inga. Cunt. Berkeley, CA : Seal Press, 1998.

Starhawk. The Fifth Sacred Thing. New York : Bantam, 1993.

Stein, Diane. A Woman's I Ching. Freedom, CA : The Crossing Press, 1997.

Waldherr, Kris. The Book of Goddesses : A Celebration of the Divine Feminine. New York, Abrams, 2006.

WHO ARE the MOON DIVAS?

LARA
IRENE
VESTA

DEVA
IRENE
MUNAY

A.K.A. FREYJA
VALKYRIE
I grew up in the deep woods of Wimer in Southern Oregon, the child of homesteading hippies. My love of the world, of nature and story and community has been nurtured in all of my transitions: marriage and mothering, divorce and development of professional life. I hold an MFA in Fiction Writing from Pacific University, where I taught for five years. Currently I am a practicing Life Cycle Celebrant and entrepreneur specializing in supporting Women in transition. ♥

A.K.A.
DURGA
MINERVA
A seasoned world traveler, sacred healer and talented teacher of plant medicine, yoga, spiritual healing and holistic health, Deva has trained with many teachers and walked many paths, all leading to this work. She makes her home in the redwoods of Big Sur, CA, where she is currently gestating projects in both book and film form. ♥

FRIENDS and Co-conspirators since 1994!

WE ARE!

AND SO ARE YOU!

MOON: la luna, sweet rock whose force moves cycle and tide in rhythm, symbol of transformation, intuition and the feminine.

DIVA: goddess, celebrated female power with sacred essence, a feminine aspect of divinity.

MOON DIVAS ARE A VISION OF HEALING, STRENGTH AND POTENT LOVE. MOON DIVAS ARE ALL POSSIBILITY AND POTENTIAL OF A NEW STORY, WHERE ALL WOMEN LOVE THEIR BODIES, LOVE THEIR STORIES AND LOVE, WHEREVER AND HOWEVER MET, THEIR LIVES. WHEN WE TEND TO THE HEART, FIND FREEDOM AND JOY IN THE FEMININE, REVERE AND RESPECT OUR BODIES, OUR CYCLES AND DAYS AS HOLY, WE LIVE THE BEAUTY WE ARE. OBSTACLES BECOME OPPORTUNITES, TRANSITIONS BECOME TRANSFORMATION. WE ARE ALL HEALERS, ALL TEACHERS, ALL GIFTED. ALL BLESSED. MOON DIVAS ARE ALL WOMEN. ALL MEN. ALL OF US. ALL WHO LOVE.

CPSIA information can be obtained at www.ICGtesting.com
Printed in the USA
BVOW06s1846071114

373528BV00005B/8/P